Challenges of Pediatric Practice in Rural America

Editor

MARY C. OTTOLINI

PEDIATRIC CLINICS OF NORTH AMERICA

www.pediatric.theclinics.com

Consulting Editor
TINA L. CHENG

February 2025 • Volume 72 • Number 1

ELSEVIER

1600 John F. Kennedy Boulevard • Suite 1800 • Philadelphia, Pennsylvania, 19103-2899

http://www.theclinics.com

THE PEDIATRIC CLINICS OF NORTH AMERICA Volume 72, Number 1
February 2025 ISSN 0031-3955, ISBN-13: 978-0-443-29582-9

Editor: Kerry Holland
Developmental Editor: Anirban Mukherjee

The Pediatric Clinics of North America (ISSN 0031-3955) is published bimonthly by Elsevier Inc., 360 Park Avenue South, New York, NY 10010-1710. Months of issue are February, April, June, August, October, and December. Periodicals postage paid at New York, NY and additional mailing offices. Subscription prices are $299.00 per year (US individuals), $380.00 per year (Canadian individuals), $453.00 per year (international individuals), $100.00 per year (US students and residents), $100.00 per year (Canadian students and residents), and $165.00 per year (international residents and students). For institutional access pricing please contact Customer Service via the contact information below. To receive students/resident rare, orders must be accompanied by name of affiliated institution, date of term, and the signature of program/residency coordinator on institution letterhead. Orders will be billed at individual rate until proof of status is received. Foreign air speed delivery is included in all *Clinics* subscription prices. All prices are subject to change without notice. Orders, claims, and journal inquiries: Please visit our Support Hub page https://service.elsevier.com for assistance.

Reprints. For copies of 100 or more, of articles in this publication, please contact the Commercial Reprints Department, Elsevier Inc., 360 Park Avenue South, New York, NY 10010-1710. Tel.: 212-633-3874; Fax: 212-633-3820; E-mail: reprints@elsevier.com.

The Pediatric Clinics of North America is also published in Spanish by McGraw-Hill Inter-americana Editores S.A., Mexico City, Mexico; in Portuguese by Riechmann and Affonso Editores, Rua Comandante Coelho 1085, CEP 21250, Rio de Janeiro, Brazil; and in Greek by Althayia SA, Athens, Greece.

The Pediatric Clinics of North America is covered in *MEDLINE/PubMed (Index Medicus), Excerpta Medica, Current Contents, Current Contents/Clinical Medicine, Science Citation Index, ASCA, ISI/BIOMED*, and *BIOSIS*.

Printed in the United States of America.

JOURNAL TITLE: Pediatric Clinics of North America
ISSUE: 72.1

PROGRAM OBJECTIVE

The goal of the *Pediatric Clinics of North America* is to keep practicing physicians and residents up to date with current clinical practice in pediatrics by providing timely articles reviewing the state-of-the-art in patient care.

TARGET AUDIENCE

All practicing pediatricians, physicians, and healthcare professionals who provide patient care to pediatric patients.

LEARNING OBJECTIVES

Upon completion of this activity, participants will be able to:

1. Review the challenges and inequity in rural America's access to care for youth.
2. Discuss various tools for improving access to subspecialty care among rural children.
3. Recognize pediatric clinicians can use existing tools and resources to optimize the care of pediatric injuries in rural environments.

ACCREDITATIONS

Physician Credit

The Elsevier Office of Continuing Medical Education (EOCME) is accredited by the Accreditation Council for Continuing Medical Education (ACCME) to provide continuing medical education for physicians.

The EOCME designates this journal-based activity for a maximum of 12 *AMA PRA Category 1 Credit*(s)™. Physicians should claim only the credit commensurate with the extent of their participation in the activity.

All other healthcare professionals requesting continuing education credit for this journal-based activity will be issued a certificate of participation.

ABP Maintenance of Certification Credit

Successful completion of this CME activity, which includes participation in the activity and individual assessment of and feedback to the learner, enables the learner to earn up to 12 MOC points in the American Board of Pediatrics' (ABP) Maintenance of Certification (MOC) program. It is the CME activity provider's responsibility to submit learner completion information to ACCME for the purpose of granting ABP MOC credit.

DISCLOSURE OF RELEVANT FINANCIAL RELATIONSHIPS

The EOCME assesses conflict of interest with its instructors, faculty, planners, and other individuals who are in a position to control the content of CME activities. All relevant conflicts of interest that are identified are thoroughly vetted by EOCME for fair balance, scientific objectivity, and patient care recommendations. EOCME is committed to providing its learners with CME activities that promote improvements or quality in healthcare and not a specific proprietary business or a commercial interest.

The authors and editors listed below have identified no financial relationships or relationships to products or devices they have with ineligible companies related to the content of this CME activity: Ahlam K. Abuawad, PhD; Rudaina Banihani, MD; Krista Birnie, MD; James C. Bohnhoff, MD, MS; Rachel M.A. Brown, MBBS, MRCPsych, FACPsych; Tina L. Cheng, MD, MPH; Paige Terrien Church, MD; Rushika Conroy, MD, MS; Rachel Criswell, MD, MS; Tyler DeAngelis, BA; Brenda Eskenazi, MA, PhD; Mary E. Fallat, MD; Michael Ferguson, MBBS, MBTeach; Abby F. Fleisch, MD, MPH; Kelsey Gleason, ScD, MS; Carrie Gordon, MD; Kenneth W. Gow, MD; Kathleen Grene, MD, MPH; Kari R. Harris, MD; Allison Holmes, MD, MPH; Jeffrey Holmes, MD; Celia Jewell, RN, MPH; Yvonne Jonk, PhD; Margaret R. Karagas, PhD; Jonathan E. Kohler, MD; Jonathan Samuel Litt, MD; Misty Melendi, MD; Ana M. Mora, MD, PhD; Michael Msall, MD; Anne M. Mullin, BS; Heidi O'Connor, MS; Carol Lynn O'Dea, MD; Valerie O'Hara, DO; Mary C. Ottolini, MD, MPH, MEd; Kristin Reese, MD; Jill Rinehart, MD, FAAP; Lisa B. Rokoff, PhD; Katie Senechal, MPH; Rachel A. Umoren, MBBCh, MS; Genevieve Whiting, MD; Matthew Workman, MD, MPH, FAAP; Brian Youth, MD, FAAP; Allison Zanno, MD; Erika Ziller, PhD

The authors and editors listed below have identified financial relationships or relationships to products or devices they have with ineligible companies related to the content of this CME activity:
Rushika Conroy, MD, MS: *Speaker*: Rhythm Pharmaceuticals, Inc. GOLD Academy

Valerie O'Hara, DO: *Speaker*: Novo Nordisk

The planning committee and staff listed below have identified no financial relationships or relationships to products or devices they have with ineligible companies related to the content of this CME activity:

Kerry Holland; Shyamala Kavikumaran; Michelle Littlejohn; Patrick J. Manley; Anirban Mukherjee

UNAPPROVED/OFF-LABEL USE DISCLOSURE

The EOCME requires CME faculty to disclose to the participants:

1. When products or procedures being discussed are off-label, unlabelled, experimental, and/or investigational (not US Food and Drug Administration [FDA] approved); and
2. Any limitations on the information presented, such as data that are preliminary or that represent ongoing research, interim analyses, and/or unsupported opinions. Faculty may discuss information about pharmaceutical agents that is outside of FDA-approved labelling. This information is intended solely for CME and is not intended to promote off-label use of these medications. If you have any questions, contact the medical affairs department of the manufacturer for the most recent prescribing information.

TO ENROLL

To enroll in the *Pediatric Clinics of North America* Continuing Medical Education program, call customer service at 1-800-654-2452 or sign up online at https://www.pediatric.theclinics.com/cme/home. The CME program is available to subscribers for an additional annual fee of USD 313.00.

METHOD OF PARTICIPATION

In order to claim credit, participants must complete the following:

1. Complete enrolment as indicated above.
2. Read the activity.
3. Complete the CME Test and Evaluation. Participants must achieve a score of 70% on the test. All CME Tests and Evaluations must be completed online.

In order to claim MOC points, participants must complete the following:

1. Complete steps listed above for claiming CME credit
2. Provide your specialty board ID#, birth date (MM/DD), and attestation.
3. Online MOC submission is only available for the American Board of pediatrics' (ABP) Maintenance of Certification (MOC) program

CME INQUIRIES/SPECIAL NEEDS

For all CME inquiries or special needs, please contact elsevierCME@elsevier.com.

Contributors

CONSULTING EDITOR

TINA L. CHENG, MD, MPH
BK Rachford Professor and Chair of Pediatrics, University of Cincinnati, Director, Cincinnati Children's Research Foundation, Chief Medical Officer, Cincinnati Children's Hospital Medical Center, Cincinnati, Ohio, USA

EDITOR

MARY C. OTTOLINI, MD, MPH, MEd
George W. Hallett MD Chair, Department of Pediatrics, The Barbara Bush Children's Hospital at Maine Medical Center, Chief, MaineHealth Children's Health Service Line, Portland, Maine, USA

AUTHORS

AHLAM K. ABUAWAD, PhD
Postdoctoral Fellow, Department of Epidemiology, Geisel School of Medicine, Children's Environmental Health and Disease Prevention Research Center at Dartmouth, Hanover, New Hampshire, USA

RUDAINA BANIHANI, MD
Associate Professor, Department of Neonatology, Sunnybrook Health Sciences Centre, Toronto, Ontario, Canada

KRISTA BIRNIE, MD
Pediatric Hospitalist, Department of Pediatrics, Seattle Children's Hospital, Seattle, Washington, USA

JAMES C. BOHNHOFF, MD, MS
Assistant Professor of Pediatrics, Tufts University School of Medicine, Boston, Massachusetts, USA; Physician Investigator, MaineHealth Pediatrics, Westbrook, Maine, USA

RACHEL M.A. BROWN, MBBS, MRCPysch, FACPysch
Professor and Chair, Department of Psychiatry and Behavioral Sciences, University of Kansas School of Medicine - Wichita, Wichita, Kansas, USA

PAIGE TERRIEN CHURCH, MD
Assistant Professor, Department of Neonatology, Beth Israel Deaconess Medical Center, Boston, Massachusetts, USA

RUSHIKA CONROY, MD, MS
Director, Pediatric Obesity Program, MaineHealth Weight Management, Maine Health, South Portland, Maine, USA; Pediatric Endocrinologist, Maine Health, Portland, Maine, USA

RACHEL CRISWELL, MD, MS
Adjunct Professor, Department of Epidemiology, Geisel School of Medicine, Children's Environmental Health and Disease Prevention Research Center at Dartmouth, Hanover, New Hampshire, USA; Assistant Professor, Tufts University School of Medicine, Boston, Massachusetts, USA; Attending Physician, Skowhegan Family Medicine, Redington-Fairview General Hospital, Skowhegan, Maine, USA

TYLER DEANGELIS, BA
Graduate Assistant, Department of Public Health, Muskie School of Public Service, University of Southern Maine, Portland, Maine, USA

BRENDA ESKENAZI, MA, PhD
Director, Center for Environmental Research and Community Health, School of Public Health, University of California, Berkeley, Berkeley, California

MARY E. FALLAT, MD
Professor, The Hiram C. Polk, Jr., Department of Surgery, University of Louisville School of Medicine, Norton Children's Hospital, Louisville, Kentucky, USA

MICHAEL FERGUSON, MBBS, MTeach
Assistant Professor, Department of Pediatrics, Tufts University School of Medicine, Boston, Massachusetts, USA; Section of Pediatric Intensive Care, Department of Pediatrics, The Barbara Bush Children's Hospital at Maine Medical Center, Portland, Maine, USA

ABBY F. FLEISCH, MD, MPH
Associate Professor of Pediatrics, Tufts University School of Medicine, Boston, Massachusetts, USA; Center for Interdisciplinary and Population Health Research, MaineHealth Institute for Research, Westbrook; Attending Physician, Pediatric Endocrinology and Diabetes, Maine Medical Center, Portland, Maine, USA

KELSEY GLEASON, ScD, MS
Assistant Professor, Department of Biomedical and Health Sciences, University of Vermont, Burlington, Vermont, USA

CARRIE GORDON, MD
Director, Let's Go. MaineHealth Weight Management, Maine Health, South Portland, Maine, USA

KENNETH W. GOW, MD
Chief, Division of Pediatric Surgery, Stony Brook University Hospital, Stony Brook, New York, USA

KATHLEEN GRENE, MD, MPH
Resident Physician, Department of Pediatrics, Yale-New Haven Hospital, New Haven, Connecticut, USA

KARI R. HARRIS, MD, FAAP
Professor, Department of Pediatrics, University of Kansas School of Medicine - Wichita, Wichita, Kansas, USA

ALISON HOLMES, MD, MPH
Associate Professor, Department of Pediatrics, Geisel School of Medicine, Dartmouth, Dartmouth Health Children's, Lebanon, New Hampshire, USA

JEFFREY HOLMES, MD
Assistant Professor, Department of Emergency Medicine, Tufts University School of Medicine, Boston, Massachusetts, USA; Regional Director of Simulation Education, The

Hannaford Center for Safety, Innovation and Simulation, Maine Medical Center, Portland, Maine, USA

CELIA JEWELL, RN, MPH
Department of Public Health, Muskie School of Public Service, Research Associate, Policy Analyst II, Maine Rural Health Research Center, University of Southern Maine, Portland, Maine, USA

YVONNE JONK, PhD
Associate Research Professor, Department of Public Health, Muskie School of Public Service, Director, Maine Rural Health Research Center, University of Southern Maine, Portland, Maine, USA

MARGARET R. KARAGAS, PhD
Department Chair and James W. Squire Professor, Department of Epidemiology, Geisel School of Medicine, Professor of Community and Family Medicine, Director, Center for Molecular Epidemiology at Dartmouth, Director, Children's Environmental Health and Disease Prevention Research Center at Dartmouth, Hanover, Hampshire, USA

JONATHAN E. KOHLER, MD
Professor, Department of Surgery, Division of Pediatric General, Thoracic and Fetal Surgery, University of California - Davis, Sacramento, California, USA

JONATHAN SAMUEL LITT, MD
Assistant Professor, Department of Neonatology, Beth Israel Deaconess Medical Center, Boston, Massachusetts, USA

MISTY MELENDI, MD
Assistant Professor, Department of Pediatrics, Tufts University School of Medicine, Boston, Massachusetts, USA; Section of Neonatal-Perinatal Medicine, Department of Pediatrics, The Barbara Bush Children's Hospital at Maine Medical Center, Portland, Maine, USA

ANA M. MORA, MD, PhD
Assistant Researcher, Center for Environmental Research and Community Health, School of Public Health, University of California, Berkeley, California, USA

MICHAEL MSALL, MD
Professor, Department of Pediatrics, Comer Children's Hospital, Chicago, Illinois, USA

ANNE M. MULLIN, BS
MD Candidate, 2025, Tufts University School of Medicine, Boston, Massachusetts, USA

HEIDI O'CONNOR, MS
Senior Data Analyst, Department of Public Health, Muskie School of Public Service, University of Southern Maine, Portland, Maine, USA

CAROL LYNN O'DEA, MD
Assistant Professor, Department of Medicine, Geisel School of Medicine, Dartmouth, Hanover, Program Director, Pediatric Residency, Children's Hospital at Dartmouth-Hitchcock, Lebanon, New Hampshire, USA

VALERIE O'HARA, DO
Medical Director, MaineHealth Weight Management, Maine Health, South Portland, Maine, USA

KRISTIN REESE, MD
Associate Professor, Department of Pediatrics, Dartmouth Health Children's, Lebanon, New Hampshire, USA, Instructor in Pediatrics, Geisel School of Medicine, Dartmouth, Hanover, New Hampshire, USA

JILL RINEHART, MD, FAAP
Associate Professor, Department of Pediatrics, Robert J. Larner College of Medicine at the University of Vermont, Pediatric Residency Program, University of Vermont Children's Hospital, Burlington, Vermont, USA

LISA B. ROKOFF, PhD
Assistant Professor of Pediatrics, Tufts University School of Medicine, Boston, Massachusetts, USA; Environmental Epidemiology Staff Scientist, Center for Interdisciplinary and Population Health Research, MaineHealth Institute for Research, Westbrook, Maine, USA

KATIE SENECHAL, SM
Candidate, 2024, Department of Epidemiology, Harvard T.H. Chan School of Public Health, Boston, Massachusetts, USA; Center for Interdisciplinary and Population Health Research, MaineHealth Institute for Research, Westbrook, Maine, USA

RACHEL A. UMOREN, MBBCH, MS
Associate Professor, Department of Pediatrics, University of Washington, Department of Pediatrics, Seattle Children's Hospital, Seattle, Washington, USA

GENEVIEVE WHITING, MD
Assistant Professor of Pediatrics, Tufts University School of Medicine, Boston, Massachusetts, USA; Associate Medical Director, MaineHealth Pediatrics, Westbrook, Maine, USA

MATTHEW WORKMAN, MD, MPH, FAAP
General Pediatrician, Peerless Pediatrics, Cleveland, Tennessee, USA

BRIAN YOUTH, MD, FAAP
Associate Professor, Department of Pediatrics, Tufts University School of Medicine, Boston, Massachusetts, USA; Community and Rural Pediatrics Rotation Director, Past Program Director, Pediatric Residency, Maine Medical Center, The Barbara Bush Children's Hospital at Maine Medical Center, Portland, Maine, USA

ALLISON ZANNO, MD
Assistant Professor, Department of Pediatrics, Tufts University School of Medicine, Boston, Massachusetts, USA; Department of Pediatrics, Section of Neonatal–Perinatal Medicine, The Barbara Bush Children's Hospital at Maine Medical Center, Portland, Maine, USA

ERIKA ZILLER, PhD
Associate Professor, Health Services Research Center, Larner College of Medicine, University of Vermont, Burlington, Vermont, USA

Contents

Foreword: Children in Rural America: Persistent Health Disparities xv

Tina L. Cheng

Preface: Rural Pediatric Health Care: A Century of Challenges and a Millennium of Opportunities xvii

Mary C. Ottolini

Overall Health Status of Rural Children and Associations with Child Poverty 1

Matthew Workman

Children living in rural areas have a shorter life expectancy and suffer from worse health outcomes compared with their urban counterparts. This disparity is highlighted by higher rates of perinatal conditions, mental and behavioral disorders, obesity, oral health, and other issues. Significant gaps in preventative health measures further exacerbate this. The root cause of these disparities can be traced back to the historic poverty experienced by rural communities. To address these health disparities, comprehensive solutions are needed to address the fundamental causes of child health disparities amidst pervasive poverty.

Treatment of Pediatric Obesity in Rural Settings: Identifying and Overcoming Barriers to Care 11

Rushika Conroy, Carrie Gordon, and Valerie O'Hara

The purpose of this study is to review the current data regarding implementing pediatric obesity treatment recommendations in rural areas. Data considering barriers to care, challenges as well as opportunities, including leveraging telemedicine, provider training, e-consults to improve pediatric obesity care are provided. Given the pediatric obesity prevalence, particularly in rural settings, a multipronged approach is needed to provide equitable access to vital care. This requires continued advocacy to address barriers, including coverage of treatments, improving broadband in rural areas, and educating patients and providers to decrease bias and stigma.

Challenges and Opportunities of Pediatric Mental Health Practice in Rural America 19

Kari R. Harris and Rachel M.A. Brown

Youth living in Rural America have increased rates of mental illness and inadequate resources to address their mental health concerns. Programs and systems are currently available to build capacity in pediatric clinicians to care for youth with mental illness and to recruit and support rural clinicians. Such programs should continue to be supported with federal and state funding and additional novel programs aimed at addressing the youth mental health crisis in North America should be developed and funded.

Reimagining Neonatal Follow-Up: An Equitable Model of Care Emphasizing Family and Child Function **93**

Paige Terrien Church, Rudaina Banihani, Jonathan Samuel Litt, and Michael Msall

This review of the history of neonatal follow-up identifies the challenges, inequity in access to care and the inequity in care delivery. It also reviews the outcomes of prematurity with a focus on common outcomes and those outcomes identified by parents as important. It assimilates the evidence around various models of care to model a program that provides care in all environments (rural and urban), leveraging local resources in collaboration with academic centers to provide greater equity in care delivery and an emphasis on function, rather than data collection.

Tools for Improving Access to Subspecialty Care Among Rural Children **111**

Genevieve Whiting and James C. Bohnhoff

Children living in rural areas encounter unique, significant barriers to the receipt of health care, including pediatric specialty care. In this article, the authors review these barriers and evaluate the advantages and limitations of various access tools intended to better connect children to specialty care. They highlight the potential of some access tools to increase rural primary care physicians' skill and involvement in their patient care, but also the risks of increasing rural primary care providers' workload and responsibilities without increasing their resources. They contextualize these benefits and risks within the quintuple aims advanced by the Institute of Healthcare Improvement.

Pediatric Telemedicine Consults to Improve Access to Intensive Care in Rural Environments **123**

Rachel A. Umoren and Krista Birnie

Recent advances in telehealth adoption prompted by the COVID-19 pandemic have highlighted the potential for improved intensive care outcomes through implementing pediatric telehealth in rural and remote settings. Telemedicine consults can be used in a variety of intensive care scenarios including procedural support, resuscitation, specialty consults, and transport. Telemedicine consults for pediatric care in rural environments improve access, cost-effectiveness, and family-centeredness. Challenges to adopting telemedicine consults for intensive care unit level care include issues around training, technology, resource allocation, and attention to how implementation exacerbate or improve health disparities.

Innovative Technology to Improve Simulation Access for Rural Clinicians **133**

Allison Zanno, Jeffrey Holmes, Michael Ferguson, and Misty Melendi

Rural pediatric clinicians face barriers to accessing health care simulation, an educational standard to prepare for high-acuity, low-occurrence (HALO) events. Simulation is typically accessible in urban academic medical centers, as it is resource-intensive owing to the necessary equipment and expertise needed to implement training. Rural hospitals face geographic and financial barriers to providing simulation training. Paradoxically, rural clinicians may benefit from additional training owing to

infrequent clinical HALO events in rural centers. Emerging simulation modalities, including mobile simulation, telesimulation, and extended reality, offer more accessible simulation alternatives for rural clinicians, addressing geographic and financial gaps in access.

Preparing Residents for Rural Practice and Advocacy: The Experiences of Three Residency Training Programs in the Northeast United States (2009–2023) **151**

Brian Youth, Carol Lynn O'Dea, and Jill Rinehart

Residents that are exposed to rural practice during their training may be more likely to consider working in rural settings after training, whether that be in primary or specialty care. The authors describe 3 programs in northern New England that have had rural rotations and opportunities for residents for decades, and discuss curricular similarities and differences, and workforce outcomes postresidency. In addition, they share a collaborative curriculum and approach to advocacy that brings residents together to share ideas and projects to learn from each other.

PEDIATRIC CLINICS OF NORTH AMERICA

FORTHCOMING ISSUES

April 2025
Social Media and Pediatric Mental Health
Paul E. Weigle and Erin L. Belfort, *Editors*

June 2025
Recognizing and Responding to Child Maltreatment
Allison M. Jackson, *Editor*

August 2025
A Practical Guide to Newborn Medicine
Kelsey Ryan and Robert M. Kliegman, *Editors*

RECENT ISSUES

December 2024
Innovative Approaches to Addressing Pediatric Mental Health
Robert T. Ammerman and Craig Erickson, *Editors*

October 2024
Pediatric Obesity: Causes, Prevention, and Treatment
Gitanjali Srivastava and Eliana M. Perrin, *Editors*

August 2024
Adolescent Medicine: Important Updates after the COVID-19 Pandemic
Renata Arrington Sanders and Errol L. Fields, *Editors*

Foreword

Children in Rural America: Persistent Health Disparities

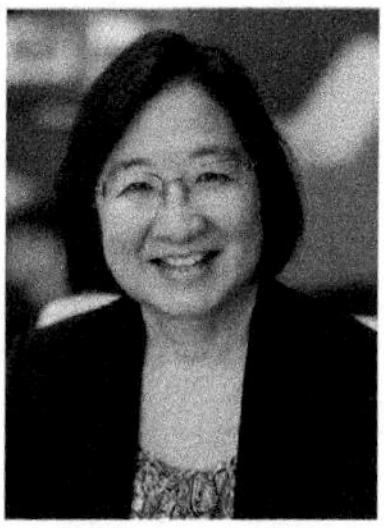

Tina L. Cheng, MD, MPH
Consulting Editor

According to the US Census Bureau, approximately 20% of Americans live in rural areas.[1] It is estimated that 12 million American children live in rural areas, with rural areas having disproportionate rates of poverty.[2] The Census Bureau's urban areas comprise a densely settled core of census blocks that meet minimum housing unit density and/or population density requirements. The territory must encompass at least 2000 housing units or have a population of at least 5000. Rural encompasses all population, housing, and territory not included within an urban area.

There are persistent and growing rural-urban health disparities. During the past three decades, mortality patterns have shifted from greater urban mortality to a "rural mortality penalty."[3,4] During this time, certain place-based measures, including race, education, income, poverty, and rurality, have been consistently associated with higher mortality rates. The direct and interacting effects of these measures are complex, but the magnitude of the high-poverty rural mortality penalty has become more important.[4] This issue of *Pediatric Clinics of North America* discusses disparities in childhood morbidity, including obesity, mental health, and injuries, demonstrating a "high-poverty rural morbidity penalty."

Poor access to care starting with prenatal care likely contributes to the rural morbidity and mortality penalty. Maternity wards and pediatric units are less profitable than adult beds. Finances and workforce challenges have contributed to closures.[5,6] It is estimated that more than half of US rural counties have no obstetric services.[6] The American Hospital Association survey found that from 2008 to 2018 pediatric inpatient units decreased by 19.1% and pediatric inpatient unit beds decreased by 11.8%, with rural areas seeing the largest decreases.[5] It was estimated that one-quarter of US children experienced an increase in distance to their nearest pediatric inpatient unit. Distance to travel for pediatric subspecialty care varies by subspecialty with

Pediatr Clin N Am 72 (2025) xv–xvi
https://doi.org/10.1016/j.pcl.2024.09.007

an estimated 1 million to 39 million children (2%–53%) residing 80 miles or more from a pediatric subspecialist and eleven subspecialties with one or fewer subspecialists per 100,000 children across hospital referral regions.[7]

This issue of *Pediatric Clinics of North America* calls attention to the challenges for children living in rural communities and that "place matters." Importantly, it outlines innovative solutions to address some of these challenges to ensure all children and adolescents thrive.

Tina L. Cheng, MD, MPH
Cincinnati Children's Hospital
Medical Center
University of Cincinnati
Cincinnati Children's Research Foundation
3333 Burnet Avenue, MLC 3016
Cincinnati, OH 45229-3026, USA

E-mail address:
Tina.cheng@cchmc.org

REFERENCES

1. US Census Bureau. Nation's urban and rural populations shift following 2020 census, December 29,2022. Available at: https://www.census.gov/newsroom/press-releases/2022/urban-rural-populations.html#:~:text=The%20rural%20population%20%E2%80%94%20the%20population,of%20changes%20to%20the%20criteria. Accessed September 10, 2024.
2. Probst JC, Barker JC, Enders A, et al. Current state of child health in rural America: how context shapes children's health. J Rural Health 2018;34(Suppl 1):s3–12. Epub 2016 Sep 28. PMID: 27677973; PMCID: PMC5373918.
3. Cosby AG, McDoom-Echebiri MM, James W, et al. Growth and persistence of place-based mortality in the United States: the rural mortality penalty. Am J Public Health 2019;109(1):155–62. Epub 2018 Nov 29. PMID: 30496008; PMCID: PMC6301407.
4. Cosby AG, Neaves TT, Cossman RE, et al. Preliminary evidence for an emerging nonmetropolitan mortality penalty in the United States. Am J Public Health 2008; 98(8):1470–2. Epub 2008 Jun 12. PMID: 18556611; PMCID: PMC2446448.
5. Cushing AM, Bucholz EM, Chien AT, et al. Availability of pediatric inpatient services in the United States. Pediatrics 2021;148(1):e2020041723. Epub 2021 Jun 14. PMID: 34127553; PMCID: PMC8642812.
6. US Government Accountability Office. Availability of hospital-based obstetric care in rural areas. 2022. Available at: https://www.gao.gov/assets/gao-23-105515.pdf. Accessed September 10, 2024.
7. Turner A, Ricketts T, Leslie LK. Comparison of number and geographic distribution of pediatric subspecialists and patient proximity to specialized care in the US between 2003 and 2019. JAMA Pediatr 2020;174(9):852–60. PMID: 32421165; PMCID: PMC7235911.

Preface

Rural Pediatric Health Care: A Century of Challenges and a Millennium of Opportunities

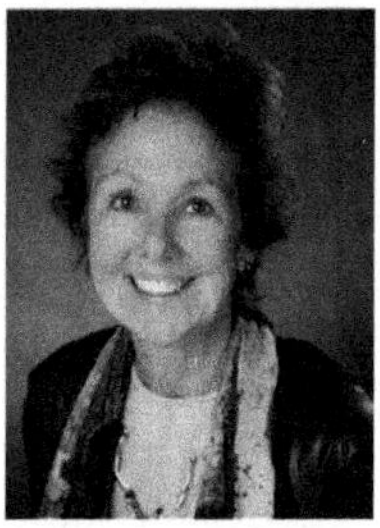

Mary C. Ottolini, MD, MPH, MEd
Editor

Prior to moving to Maine, the most rural state in the nation, I did not have much experience with rural pediatric health care, other than anecdotes from my mother. My mother was born in rural Iowa in 1925 and told stories of being transported by a horse and sleigh through a blizzard at the age of four for a life-saving chest tube to treat her pneumonia and having a pitchfork accidentally poked through her foot while working in the hayloft at age ten. These stories exemplify some of the rural pediatric health care challenges that still exist a century later, such as poverty, physician scarcity, inadequate transportation, and agriculture-related trauma.

I spent the first 35 years of my pediatric career practicing primary care and hospital medicine in urban underserved communities situated in large cities. Although poverty, race, and adverse social determinants of health are strong drivers of inequities in health care delivery among both urban and rural children, geographic isolation poses a disproportionate barrier to a healthy childhood in rural communities across the United States.

In this issue of *Pediatric Clinics of North America* authors with decades of experience practicing pediatrics and caring for children in rural settings discuss the persistent challenges patients and their health care providers encounter, as well as exciting mitigation strategies suing training and technology. The article in this issue entitled "Overall Health Status of Rural Children and Associations with Child Poverty" provides an overview of the health status of children and health care delivery in rural America. Subsequent articles describe the maladies that rural children disproportionately experience, such as obesity ("Treatment of Pediatric Obesity in Rural Settings: Identifying and Overcoming Barriers to Care"), mental illness ("Challenges and Opportunities of Pediatric Mental Health Practice in Rural America"), opiate exposure ("Opioid Use

Pediatr Clin N Am 72 (2025) xvii–xix
https://doi.org/10.1016/j.pcl.2024.09.002

Disorder and Neonatal Opioid Withdrawal Syndrome in Rural Environments"), traumatic injuries ("Optimizing the Care of Pediatric Injuries in Rural Environments"), and exposure to toxic environmental hazards ("A Call for Pediatric Clinicians to Address Environmental Health Concerns in Rural Settings"). Other articles describe obstacles to access health care, such as ambulance deserts ("Social Vulnerability of Pediatric Populations living in Ambulance Deserts") and closure of obstetric and newborn units in rural hospitals ("Innovative Technology to Improve Simulation Access for Rural Clinicians"). These health care delivery challenges are problematic for all rural children, but especially for those with medical complexity. "Reimagining Neonatal Follow-Up: An Equitable Model of Care Emphasizing Family and Child Function" is therefore devoted to describing the evolution of rural health care delivery for medically complex newborns after discharge.

There is hope on the horizon, however, based upon programs aimed at better understanding the needs and strengths of rural communities. In "Tools for Improving Access to Subspecialty Care Among Rural Children," the authors describe how technology can offer patients and primary care providers access to specialty care in the form of outreach clinics, telemedicine, and eConsults. Telemedicine as an option for specialty consultation and coaching in rural delivery rooms and emergency departments to resuscitate and stabilize critically ill patients is covered in "Pediatric Telemedicine Consults to Improve Access to Intensive Care Unit Care in Rural Environments." New simulation training modalities, such as telesimulation and virtual/augmented reality, as described in "Innovative Technology to Improve Simulation Access for Rural Clinicians," provide opportunities for rural health care teams to train in preparation for HALO (High Acuity Low Occurrence) events. Team simulation training can supplement limited real-life opportunities to practice resuscitation skills for infants and children. This training, coupled with expert coaching provided virtually from PICU and NICU attendings in tertiary care children's hospitals, has the potential to significantly enhance rural team confidence and patient outcomes.

In addition to innovative methods to augment the expertise of current rural providers and health care teams, we would be remiss not to address developing the rural pediatric workforce of the future. "Preparing Residents for Rural Practice and Advocacy: The Experiences of Three Residency Training Programs in the Northeast United States (2009–2023)" describes successful graduate medical education programs focused on attracting and training the rural pediatricians of the future. I have seen firsthand how investment in high-quality medical school and residency programs focused on providing pediatric training in rural practices can pay huge dividends in graduates choosing to join those practices and committing to spending a career in a rural community. Although many challenges persist in delivering equitable pediatric health care delivery in rural settings, the outlook is optimistic if we are willing to invest in building the healthiest communities in America for rural children.

DISCLOSURES

The author has no conflicts of interest.

Mary C. Ottolini, MD, MPH, MEd
Department of Pediatrics
The Barbara Bush Children's Hospital
at Maine Medical Center
4908 Coloumbe Family Tower
22 Bramhall Street
Portland, ME 04102, USA

E-mail address:
Mary.ottolini@Mainehealth.org

Overall Health Status of Rural Children and Associations with Child Poverty

Matthew Workman, MD, MPH, FAAP*

KEYWORDS

• Rural children • Poverty • Disparity • Preventative health

KEY POINTS

- There is a historic gap between the health of rural children and their urban counterparts that remains today.
- This gap is highlighted and exacerbated by the increased rates of poverty in rural children.
- Rural children experience higher rates of a multitude of health conditions, including obesity, behavioral disorders, overall disability, and alcohol/drug abuse.
- Rural children are less likely to receive recommended preventative medical and dental care and have lower immunization rates than urban children.
- Geographic, cultural, and economic factors play a significant role in the persistence of health disparities experienced by rural children and adolescents.

INTRODUCTION

Rural children experience worse health outcomes than urban children.[1] This disparity is further widened when controlling for the poverty rate. Rural residents recorded smaller gains in life expectancy from 1990 to 2014 than their urban counterparts, resulting in an increased rural-urban disparity in life expectancy.[2] Economic factors, geographic isolation, and inadequate health care infrastructure contribute to widening the gap between rural and urban children. Despite efforts to address these challenges, rural communities continue to struggle with higher rates of persistent poverty and limited access to available health services.[3]

HISTORY

After the turn of the twentieth century, great strides were made in public health; through efforts such as modern sanitation, water and sewage facilities, and modern public health services, urban health improved by leaps and bounds throughout the early

Peerless Pediatrics, 1060 Peerless Crossing Suite 100, Cleveland, TN 37312, USA
* Corresponding author.
E-mail addresses: Mworkman@Peerlesspediatrics.com; workmanm00@gmail.com

Pediatr Clin N Am 72 (2025) 1–10
https://doi.org/10.1016/j.pcl.2024.07.021 **pediatric.theclinics.com**
0031-3955/25/

twentieth century. By the 1920s, a stark contrast regarding health between urban and rural populations began to develop. People living in rural areas saw a greater frequency of infectious and preventable diseases, including dysentery, typhoid, hookworm, and malaria. Rural children also shared a disproportionate burden of congenital disabilities, with many sources placing the rate as 5% to 20% higher among rural youth. Rural child mortality was far higher than that among urban populations of the time. Geographic conditions, including distance from medical care, significantly contributed to this disparity. Still, general poverty, inadequate public health programs, and lagging sanitation programs were the most significant contributors to childhood morbidity and mortality in rural areas of the United States during the early 20th century.[4]

Through the mid-1900s, there were fantastic gains in public health, with a sharp decrease in rates of malaria through the use of insecticides and improvement of malarial land (swamp drainage), decreasing rates of hookworm infestation through widespread adoption of indoor bathrooms and running water, and a sharp decrease in rates of pellagra with the introduction of niacin-fortified foods. With improvements in sanitation and public health services, rural health continued to improve throughout the middle to late 1900s. Yet, rural children lagged and continue to lag behind their urban counterparts on many vital measures, including overall morbidity and mortality, access to care, chronic disease burden, mental and behavioral health, and preventative health.[4]

The gap between rural and urban children has decreased and changed over time but persists. This article attempts to delve further into current trends and disparities and help identify some strengths to build upon and challenges for pediatric clinicians and others working with children and adolescents living in rural areas.

DEFINITIONS

Rural Defined

Most often, rurality is defined at the county level. The most used dichotomous measure is from the Office of Management and Budget (OMB), which delineates counties as either metropolitan or nonmetropolitan. A metropolitan or urban county is a county that contains a population cluster with more than 50,000 persons, and a county is considered nonmetropolitan or rural if it does not.[3] This county-level delineation undercounts many rural populations, especially in states where counties encompass a large geographic area. The term rural has multiple definitions, typically based on policy or research needs. Throughout this article, the term rural, when used as a designation, will typically be based on county or zip code data (ZCTAs), or it will be clearly defined within context.

Rural Children Defined

Utilizing definitions of rurality provided by the Department of Health and Human Services, the US Food and Drug Administration, the American Academy of Pediatrics, and the US Dept of Agriculture (USDA), approximately 11.8 million children and adolescents lived in rural areas as of 2018. The demographic composition of rural children and adolescents shows a predominance of non-Hispanic white children (71.8%), with Hispanic (11.9%), non-Hispanic Black children (9.4%), Asian/Pacific Islander (0.9%), and other (6.1%) comprising the remainder.[3]

BACKGROUND

Economic Characteristics of Rural America

The economies of rural counties are more sensitive to economic pressure and trends that affect their largest industries. Although thought of as primarily agrarian communities, according to the USDA most rural counties rely on more than agriculture as a driver of local economies. Twenty percent of rural counties are considered farming-dependent; around 10% depend on mining and gas operations, and a further 20% depend on manufacturing as a source of employment and economic stimuli. The remaining rural counties have greater economic diversity and do not rely on 1 major industry.[5] Rural communities lagged behind their urban counterparts from 2011 to 2018. Of the top 100 counties with the highest childhood poverty rates in 2014, 95 were rural.[3] Manyof these counties also have a large minority population. There is an over-representation of adverse socio-demographic indicators; these include persistent child poverty, high unemployment rates, and low rates of education. Counties where the rates of children living in poverty have exceeded 20% for the past 30 years, known as persistent child poverty counties, are concentrated in specific regions, including the Deep South, the Southwest, the US-Mexican border, central Appalachia, the Central Valley of California, and the American Indian Reservations of the Northern Plains.[3]

Economic Characteristics of Rural Children

Rural children are more likely than their adult counterparts to live in poverty. Twenty-four percent of children in rural areas live in poverty, compared with 17% of adults.[6] The gap between urban and rural children is inversely correlated with age. In 2019, according to the USDA, the most significant difference between rural and urban poverty rates was for children under 5 (24% in rural areas and 17.3% in urban areas). Children between the ages of 5 and 18 still maintained a significant gap (21.1% in rural areas and 16.1% in urban areas), but the gap continues to close among working age (18–64 years of age) and is statistically nonexistent in seniors (over 65 years of age), with 10.3% of senior is rural areas living in poverty and 9.3% of seniors in urban areas living in poverty.[5]

Race is an independent variable regarding poverty in rural areas and is correlated with increased poverty in children and an increase in poverty persistence for multiple generations. As of 2019, for all ages, rural African Americans/Blacks had the highest incidence of poverty at 30.7%. Rural Native Americans/Alaska Natives held the second highest rate at 29.6%. Rural Hispanics had the third highest poverty rate at 21.7%, while rural Caucasians/Whites had a rate of 13.3%; 51.1% of African American children living in rural counties live below the federal poverty level compared with 37.2% of African American children living in urban counties[5] **Table 1**.

CURRENT EVIDENCE

Overall Health

Rurality is a known independent risk factor associated with an increased risk of overall morbidity and mortality.[7] This increased risk has been shown across the full spectrum of pediatrics.[8] Rural children and adolescents are at a greater risk of being affected by neonatal-abstinence syndrome, having lower rates of completed childhood vaccines, having visual, hearing, or learning disabilities, being obese, engaging in high-risk sexual activity, engaging in alcohol and illicit drug use, and being diagnosed with a mental, behavioral, or developmental disorder.[2,3,9]

Access

Access to a pediatrician or pediatric provider has been well documented as lacking in rural areas, but the contrast remains stark. Many factors affect health care access for rural children, including insurance coverage, provider workforce, and travel burdens/

Table 1
Demographics of rural and nonrural children[a,b]

	Rural[c], %	Nonrural, %
Overall, n (%)	15,166,752 (19.5)	62,721,267 (80.5)
Age		
0–1 y	9.6	9.8
2–5 y	20.0	20.7
6–10 y	26.4	26.2
11–14 y	21.7	21.5
15–18 y	22.4	21.8
Sex		
Male	51.4	51.1
Female	48.6	48.9
Race/ethnicity		
Non-Hispanic White	70.4	46.0
Non-Hispanic Black	9.0	14.5
Hispanic	12.8	27.9
American Indian or Alaska Native	2.3	0.4
Asian	1.1	5.7
Other	4.4	5.4
Health insurance		
None	6.1	4.9
Private	55.3	61.0
Public	42.9	37.5
Income to federal poverty level		
0%–50% FPL	10.6	8.4
51%–100% FPL	11.8	10.0
101%–150% FPL	12.8	10.9
151%–200% FPL	11.8	9.8
>200% FPL	53.0	60.8

[a] Estimates obtained through the 2019 American Community Survey 5-year estimates administered by IPUMS. Source: Ruggles S, Flood S, Foster S, et al. IPUMS USA: Version 11.0 [dataset]. Minneapolis, Minnesota: IPUMS, 2021. doi:https://doi.org/10.18128/D010.V11.0.

[b] IPUMS defines geographic areas using the variable METRO and with the following approach: "METRO indicates whether the household resided within a metropolitan area and, for households in metropolitan areas, whether the household resided within or outside of a central/principal city. In many public-use microdata samples, metropolitan and central/principal-city status is not directly identified. In such cases, IPUMS derives METRO codes based on other available geographic information, for example, county groups (CNTYGP97 and CNTYGP98) or public use microdata areas (PUMA). If a county group or PUMA lies only partially within metropolitan areas or central/principal cities, then METRO indicates that the status is indeterminable (mixed)."

[c] In this analysis, mixed was classified as rural, as the sum of the weighted percentage of rural and mixed areas defined by the IPUMS METRO variable similar to the percentages of rural population defined by other governmental agencies.[6,7]

transportation issues;[9] 84.9% of the nation's rural counties are at least partially designated as a health professional shortage area (HPSAs). Some of these areas have a rate of 22 pediatricians/family physicians per 100,000 children or 1 pediatrician/family physician per 4500 children, and 56.6% of rural counties lack a pediatrician.[3] In addition to pediatricians and family physicians, nurse practitioners (NPs)and physician assistants (PAs) play a significant role in rural pediatric primary care. But, as training for NPs and PAs continues to increase across the country, only 9% of NPs specialize in pediatrics, and even fewer PAs choose to practice in pediatrics (2.4% in general pediatrics and 1.6% in pediatric subspecialties).[10,11]

Many rural areas lack access to pediatric care, which leads to greater travel distances for families seeking primary or specialty care. Limited access to transportation options for rural families exacerbates this issue. Telemedicine has been touted as a solution to issues related to access, but barriers, including lacking broadband access and poorer digital literacy, contribute to challenges for families seeking pediatric care. Rural and urban children have similar overall rates of insurance, but the source is significantly different. In rural counties, 46.8% of children are covered by Medicaid compared with 34.9% of urban children.[3]

All-Cause Mortality

Rural infants and children experience higher rates of all-cause mortality than their urban counterparts.[2] The leading causes of infant deaths in the United States are congenital disabilities, preterm births, low birth weight, sudden infant death syndrome (SIDS), and accidental and nonaccidental trauma.[8] Rural infants share a disproportionate burden of these causes of death. Per US Centers for Disease Control and Prevention (CDC) data, the rate of infant death due to congenital disabilities was 16 per 10,000 live births in rural areas and 12 per 10,000 live births in urban areas.[8] Among older children and young adults, those living in rural areas remain particularly vulnerable. Some of the major causes of death in this age group include motor vehicle accidents, firearm-related injury, drowning, and drug overdose/poisoning.[12] Infant and child mortality rates have been shown to be higher in rural areas than in urban areas for all demographics, but Black infants and children in poor, rural communities have nearly 3 times higher mortality rates compared with those in affluent rural areas.[2]

Obesity

Based on data from the National Survey of Children's Health in 2019 and 2020, rural children were more likely than self-reported urban children to be overweight or obese (37.6% versus 32.1%).[13] Rural children were also more likely to experience food insecurity than their urban counterparts (39.6% versus 31.1%).[8] Also of note, children living below 400% of the federal poverty level (FPL) were at a greater risk of being overweight or obese regardless of rurality. This increase in rates of obesity among rural children is again seen throughout the spectrum of pediatrics. Statistically significant differences in body mass index (BMI) between rural and urban children have been shown from preschool aged children throughout the spectrum of childhood.[13] Meta-analyses have shown between 26% and 30% increased risk of obesity among school-aged children in rural areas.[14]

Mental, Behavioral, and Developmental Disorders

Disparate rates between rural children and adolescents and urban children concerning mental, behavioral, and developmental disorders (MBDDs) have been shown in some studies at the county, state, and national levels.[15,16] The most common forms of MBDDs include attention-deficit/hyperactivity disorder (ADHD), anxiety, depression, and autism spectrum disorder. Based on data from the 2016 National Survey of Children's Health, socioeconomic status is inversely correlated with MBDD risk, with children who live in lower-income households (less than 100% of the FPL) 8.2% more likely than children living in higher-income households (greater than

400% of the FPL) to have ever received a diagnosis of an MBDD (22.1% versus 13.9%).[17]

With the onset of the coronavirus disease 2019 (COVID-19) pandemic and subsequent mitigation measures, mental and behavioral health has been thrust into the spotlight. Children and adolescents bore some of the greatest burdens regarding mental and behavioral health throughout the COVID-19 pandemic and continue to have rates above prepandemic levels. Adolescents and children have experienced higher rates of anxiety and depression since the start of the COVID-19 pandemic.[13]

Although rural children and adolescents have higher rates of mental, behavioral, and developmental disorders, they are less likely than urban children and adolescents to access behavioral and developmental services.[18] Among youth with a psychiatric diagnosis visiting hospital emergency departments, rural children and adolescents were more likely to be hospitalized after controlling for clinical needs.[3] This highlights the lagging availability of effective outpatient resources for these patients.

Preventative Medicine and Immunizations

Even before the COVID-19 pandemic, rural children were less likely than their urban counterparts to have received a preventative medical or dental visit in the last 12 months, 59.6% to 66.7%, respectively. Household income is a protective factor for preventative medical and dental care in rural and urban children, but the gap in preventative care persists regardless of household income or poverty level.[19]

Recent studies show that immunizations, perhaps the most significant preventative care measure for children and adolescents, are significantly lower in rural areas.[20] Studies out of Wisconsin show rates of both human papilloma virus (HPV) vaccine uptake and completion 4% to 5% lower in rural zip codes.[21] Vaccination coverage for adolescents living in rural areas was lower compared with adolescents living in urban/suburban areas; rural adolescents had a 9.8% lower rate of at least 1 dose of HPV vaccine (68.0% versus 77.8%), a 4.5% lower rate of at least 1 dose of meningococcal conjugate (MenACWY) vaccine (85.7% versus 90.2%), and a 7.4% lower rate of 2 doses of hepatitis A vaccine.[22]

Worsening overall rates of vaccine uptake are exacerbated in rural areas where access is already an issue. During the COVID-19 pandemic, children living in rural areas or below the poverty line had a decrease in vaccine coverage at 2 years of all 7 recommended vaccines of 4 % to 5%.[23] HPV vaccine uptake also sharply declined during the COVID-19 pandemic, with rates 25% to 50% below prepandemic levels throughout 2020 and 2021.[23] Even before the COVID-19 pandemic, an increase in parental hesitancy regarding the safety and efficacy of vaccines was seen throughout the United States.[24] Worsening overall rates of vaccine uptake are exacerbated in rural areas where access is already an issue. Rural children are more likely to receive vaccines at public facilities (ie, a local health department or community health center) or through nontraditional means (community immunization pop-ups) than their urban counterparts, creating both barriers and unique opportunities.[24]

DISCUSSION

Rural children experience a disproportionate burden of adverse health outcomes, including all-cause mortality, obesity, oral health, autism spectrum disorder, ADHD, anxiety, and depression; have a higher frequency of adverse childhood events (ACEs); experience greater rates of food insecurity; and are more likely to be exposed to household dysfunction.[25] Many of the disparities discussed have their roots in rural poverty. More than 1 in every 5 children living in rural areas in the United States lives in poverty.[26] For families living in rural areas, the income inequality experienced makes it difficult to meet basic needs like food and shelter in addition to paying for health care. Poverty also exerts a significant independent effect on an individual level through increased stress markers.[26]

Physical environmental factors also play a significant role in the health of rural children. Rural areas have several disadvantages, including low walkability, limitations of public transport, fewer facilities for physical activity, and large travel distances to recreational areas, which have been implicated as environmental challenges for rural communities.[27] This also highlights the significant differences that rural communities have from one another. Physical environments are drastically different from 1 geographic region to the next. Although some solutions are replicable in rural communities, the challenges that rural Tennessee faces are different from those that rural Maine faces, which are different from the challenges that rural Alaska faces, and so on. Comprehensive solutions addressing health care and health outcome disparities experienced by rural children and adolescents must be tailored to the community's strengths and weaknesses.

Rural communities' capacity to improve their children's health is present but limited. From an economic standpoint, people in rural communities have lower access to educational opportunities, and, in turn, decreased access to high-paying jobs. In a 2013 study from the Carsey Institute, rural areas rely on what was termed middle-skill jobs that require on-the-job training or an apprenticeship. Urban areas tend to have a lower percentage of these middle-skill jobs while having a similar number of low-skill jobs and a higher number of high-skilled jobs (minimum of a bachelor's degree). This study also found that many highly skilled workers living in rural areas had lower pay than their urban colleagues.[28]

Historically, this has led to a diaspora of highly skilled workers from rural areas. This further leads to less economic investment in these areas from companies looking for highly skilled workers, perpetuating the cycle. Breaking that cycle has been the focus of many rural improvement initiatives over the past decade at the local, state, and national levels. In the author's home state of Tennessee, 1 such success story has been the partnership of the Tennessee Board of Regents and the National Rural Education Association in developing a regional approach to workforce development in 4 rural counties. With help from USDA grant funding, this partnership increased technical career awareness among kindergarten through grade 12 students and allowed graduating high school students to earn college credit and technical certifications.[6] This is 1 example of many efforts to address the economic burden on rural areas and the root causes of persistent child poverty and poor health outcomes in rural communities.

SUMMARY

Historically, children living in rural areas have faced greater challenges in health care access and infrastructure, leading to higher rates of many health issues, including overall mortality, neonatal abstinence syndrome, developmental delays, obesity, ADHD, anxiety, depression, and a multitude of other poverty-related health issues compared with children living in urban areas. Despite advancements in rural public health throughout the twentieth century, rural children remain behind their urban peers in many health indicators. Many of these disparities are rooted in rural poverty, with rural areas experiencing higher rates of persistent poverty, unemployment, and limited access to educational and job opportunities. Rural children are more likely to live in poverty, experience food insecurity, and lack adequate access to health services, including appropriate preventative care. The challenges for rural communities looking to improve the health of their youngest members include economic, environmental, and systemic factors. Efforts to address these disparities require a comprehensive approach focusing on improving economic and educational opportunities, improving health care infrastructure and access, and addressing cultural barriers to care.

CLINICS CARE POINTS

- Infant and child mortality rates have been shown to be higher in rural areas than in urban areas for all demographics.[2]
- Rural counties lag behind urban counties in regard to persistent poverty, and children are at an even greater risk of experiencing poverty than their adult counterparts.[6]
- Rural residence is associated with an increased risk of all-cause mortality and morbidity that spans the spectrum of pediatrics.[2]
- Rural children are less likely to receive recommended preventative medical and dental care and are less likely to receive recommended immunizations.[19–21]
- Rural children experience challenges regarding access to pediatric clinicians, including significant shortages of trained pediatric clinicians, insurance barriers, greater travel distances, and limited transportation options.[9]

DISCLOSURES

The author has nothing to disclose.

REFERENCES

1. National Advisory Committee. Child poverty in rural America. Washington, DC, Available at: https://www.hrsa.gov/sites/default/files/hrsa/advisory-committees/rural/publications/2015-child-poverty.pdf, 2015. (Accessed January 2024).
2. Singh GK, Daus GP, Allender M, et al. Social determinants of health in the united states: addressing major health inequality trends for the nation, 1935-2016. Int J MCH AIDS 2017;6(2):139–64.
3. Probst JC, Barker JC, Enders A, et al. Current state of child health in rural America: how context shapes children's health. J Rural Health 2018;34:3–12.
4. Brown DC, Barreca A, Clay K, et al. Health of farm children in the South, 1900-1950. Agric Hist 1979;53(1):170–87.
5. Davis JC, Cromartie J, Farrigan T, et al. Rural America at a glance: 2023 edition (Report No. EIB-261). Washington DC: US Department of Agriculture, Economic Research Service; 2023.
6. Rogers CC. "Rural children at a glance," economic information bulletin 33899, United States Department of Agriculture, *Economic Research Service*, Economic Imformation Bulletin, vol. 1, 1-6. 2005.
7. Manemann SM, St Sauver J, Henning-Smith C, et al. Rurality, death, and health-care utilization in heart failure in the community. J Am Heart Assoc 2021;10(4): e018026.
8. Ely DM, Driscoll AK. Infant mortality in the United States, 2021: data from the period linked birth/infant death file. Natl Vital Stat Rep 2023;72(11):1–19.
9. Hung P, Workman M, Mohan K, et al. Overview of rural child health. Washington D.C., USA: National Rural Health Association; 2020.
10. Morgan PA, Hooker RS. Choice of specialties among physician assistants in the United States. Health Aff 2010;29(5):887–92.

11. Freed GL, Dunham KM, Loveland-Cherry CJ, et al, Research Advisory Committee of the American Board of Pediatrics. Pediatric nurse practitioners in the United States: current distribution and recent trends in training. J Pediatr 2010;157(4): 589–93.e1.
12. Perritt KR, Hendricks KJ, Goldcamp EM. Young worker injury deaths: a historical summary of surveillance and investigative findings. Morgantown. WV US Dep Heal Hum Serv Public Heal Serv Centers Dis Control Prev Natl Inst Occup Saf Heal DHHS Publ No 2017-168 2017;1–128.
13. Crouch E, Abshire DA, Wirth MD, et al. Rural–urban differences in overweight and obesity, physical activity, and food security among children and adolescents. Prev Chronic Dis 2023;20:230136.
14. Contreras DA, Martoccio TL, Brophy-Herb HE, et al. Rural-urban differences in body mass index and obesity-related behaviors among low-income preschoolers. J Public Health 2021;43(4):e637–44.
15. Davis DW, Jawad K, Feygin Y, et al. Disparities in ADHD diagnosis and treatment by race/ethnicity in youth receiving Kentucky Medicaid in 2017. Ethn Dis 2021; 31(1):67–76.
16. Zgodic A, McLain AC, Eberth JM, et al. County-level prevalence estimates of ADHD in children in the United States. Ann Epidemiol 2023;79:56–64.
17. Cree RA, Bitsko RH, Robinson LR, et al. Health care, family, and community factors associated with mental, behavioral, and developmental disorders and poverty among children aged 2-8 Years - United States, 2016. MMWR Morb Mortal Wkly Rep 2018;67(50):1377–83. Published 2018 Dec 21.
18. Jones EAK, Mitra AK, Bhuiyan AR. Impact of COVID-19 on mental health in adolescents: a systematic review. Int J Environ Res Publ Health 2021;18(5):2470. Published 2021 Mar 3.
19. National survey of children's health impacts of the COVID-19 pandemic, HRSA Maternal and Child Health, October 2022. Available at: https://mchb.hrsa.gov/sites/default/files/mchb/data-research/National-Survey-of-Childrens-Health-Impacts-Covid19-Pandemic-508.pdf. (Accessed January 2024).
20. Walker TJ, Rodriguez SA, Vernon SW, et al. Validity and reliability of measures to assess constructs from the inner setting domain of the consolidated framework for implementation research in a pediatric clinic network implementing HPV programs. BMC Health Serv Res 2019;19(1):205.
21. Cull Weatherer A, Pritzl SL, Kerch S, et al. Current trends in HPV vaccine uptake: Wisconsin and United States, 2016-2019. Wis Med J 2021;120(1):62–5.
22. Pingali C, Yankey D, Elam-Evans LD, et al. National, regional, state, and selected local area vaccination coverage among adolescents aged 13-17 years - United States, 2020. MMWR Morb Mortal Wkly Rep 2021;70(35):1183–90. Published 2021 Sep 3.
23. Smith DL, Perkins RB. Low rates of HPV vaccination and cervical cancer screening: Challenges and opportunities in the context of the COVID-19 pandemic. Prev Med 2022;159:107070.
24. Albers AN, Thaker J, Newcomer SR. Barriers to and facilitators of early childhood immunization in rural areas of the United States: a systematic review of the literature. Prev Med Rep 2022;27:101804. Published 2022 Apr 25.
25. Kelleher KJ, Gardner W. Out of sight, out of mind - behavioral and developmental care for rural children. N Engl J Med 2017;376(14):1301–3.
26. Bettenhausen JL, Winterer CM, Colvin JD. Health and poverty of rural children: an under-researched and under-resourced vulnerable population. Acad Pediatr 2021;21(8S):S126–33.

27. Cleland V, Hughes C, Thornton L, et al. A qualitative study of environmental factors important for physical activity in rural adults. PLoS One 2015;10(11): e0140659. Published 2015 Nov 10.
28. Young J., Middle-skill jobs remain more common among rural workers, 2013, The Carsey School of Public Policy at the Scholars' Repository, 196, Carsey Institute Issue Briefs. Available at: https://scholars.unh.edu/carsey/196. (Accessed January 2024).

Treatment of Pediatric Obesity in Rural Settings

Identifying and Overcoming Barriers to Care

Rushika Conroy, MD, MS[a,b,*], Carrie Gordon, MD[a], Valerie O'Hara, DO[a]

KEYWORDS

• Pediatric • Obesity • Telemedicine • Rural • Equity

KEY POINTS

- Barriers to effective obesity care for pediatric patients living in rural settings include lack of access to treatment, limited insurance coverage, limited obesity medicine providers, weight bias and stigma as well as the lack of extensive pediatric-focused clinical obesity research.
- Ways to overcome these barriers have been implemented but challenges remain.
- Telehealth-based programs can be successful in treating pediatric obesity in rural settings.
- Further research into effective treatment of pediatric obesity in rural settings is needed.

4

INTRODUCTION

According to the World Health Organization, over 300 million children and adolescents globally have the disease of obesity, with 14.7 million in the United States. While new and effective options have been developed as adjuncts to standard obesity treatment practices, the number of children and adolescents who suffer from obesity has not declined. Numerous factors contribute, ranging from the availability of affordable nutrient-dense foods to third-party payor reimbursement for treatment. One such factor is ineffective delivery of care to those who live in areas where the disease is highly prevalent, such as areas of lower socioeconomic status and rural settings. An understanding of these factors allows us to identify barriers and develop strategies to overcome them. In doing so, the prevalence of pediatric obesity will decrease can reduce pediatric obesity prevalence, which will hopefully lead to a reduction in adult obesity prevalence and the pediatric and adult-onset comorbidities that come with the

[a] MaineHealth Weight Management, 41 Donald B Dean Drive, South Portland, ME 04106, USA;
[b] Maine Health, 887 Congress Street, Suite 300, Portland, ME 04102, USA
* Corresponding author. 41 Donald B Dean Drive, South Portland, ME 04106.
E-mail address: Rushika.conroy@mainehealth.org

Pediatr Clin N Am 72 (2025) 11–18
https://doi.org/10.1016/j.pcl.2024.07.024 **pediatric.theclinics.com**
0031-3955/25/

disease. This document highlights the current data on implementing pediatric obesity treatment in rural settings, barriers to effective care, and potential ways to overcome them.

Data from 2011 to 2012 compared to 2017 to 2020 outline that there has been an increase in obesity for children aged 2 to 5 years and for adolescents aged 12 to 19 years.[1] The trend of higher incidence of obesity, with more severe classification of obesity at younger ages compared to 12 years ago, highlights the added negative health risk for these patients.[2] The prevalence of obesity, and particularly for severe obesity (class 2 and 3), is higher for those living in rural and underserved areas, lower socioeconomic settings, and those with high-risk social determinants of health screens.[3] Flattum and colleagues[4] compared family-based preventive intervention in urban versus rural settings, finding 20% to 25% higher odds of obesity for those living in a rural setting. McDaniel and colleagues[5] reviewed current trends in the barriers of travel needed to provide care even for common pediatric medical diagnoses and found that overall, children living in rural areas traveled 4 times further for hospitalization in 2017 compared to 2002. Thirty-four million Americans live in rural communities and providing care to children living in these rural settings has unique challenges.

A full spectrum of care is required to optimally manage obesity across the lifespan. Growing research and evidence-based guidelines support that these therapies should be delivered in an empathetic and compassionate patient-centric approach. Access to care in these areas continues to be diminished and challenges for implementation and sustainability of intensive health and lifestyle behavior therapy and specialty obesity care persist.

In January of 2023, the American Academy of Pediatrics released a clinical practice guideline (CPG) for the evaluation and treatment of childhood and adolescent obesity.[6] This guideline, a massive undertaking that started with a review of 16,000 abstracts and ultimately included almost 350 articles, was a dramatic shift in the Academy's recommendations, incorporating new, effective therapies for obesity treatment and highlighting the need to choose therapies that treat obesity and its comorbidities concurrently. The recommendations consider the multifactorial causes of obesity, including the socioeconomic and racial disparities that have contributed to disease risk. They review challenges in the communication of body mass index (BMI) status in the clinical setting, some of the limitations of use of BMI, the need for improved access to medications and surgery, and the deficit of available intensive health, behavior, and lifestyle therapy (IHBLT) programs, which are intended to be the first line of care for obesity treatment in children who are at the age of 6 years or older. Authors included recommendations on evaluation of comorbid illness that align with those from other pediatric specialty societies, with some nuanced changes to optimize care in the setting of obesity.

Implementation of new CPG has historically been found to take over a decade[7,8] and can be complicated by multiple factors, including, but not limited to, guideline complexity, guideline dissemination, education, and training and clinical decision support systems.[9] Optimizing implementation of the American Academy of Pediatrics CPG recommendations for obesity evaluation and treatment in a rural setting needs to utilize a multifaceted approach, keeping evidence for how to promote practice guideline adherence in mind.

Studies have been conducted on strategies to implement obesity care to children and adolescents who live in rural settings, with many focusing on the use of telehealth following the coronavirus disease of 2019 (COVID-19) pandemic. Janicke and colleagues randomized children with obesity who reside in a rural setting to one of 3 interventions: lifestyle and behavior modification for the family; lifestyle and behavior modification for the parents only; and lifestyle modification alone for the family. The attendance during the treatment sessions peaked at 69%, while attendance during the maintenance sessions decreased to 42%. The main barrier noted for all 3 groups regarding attendance was scheduling conflicts. There was no significant improvement in weight or BMI z-score in any of the groups.[10] Hosseini and Yilmaz[11] conducted a feasibility study examining a telehealth intervention for families in rural Pennsylvania. They found that there was a mix between families who prefer in-person visits and those who prefer telehealth visits, but no differences in BMI change were noted between groups. A study using a program called IAmHealthy found family satisfaction with the telehealth aspect of this 6 month intensive behavioral obesity intervention. The program is composed of 15 hours of didactic family group sessions and 11 hours of health coaching for the family.[12] There had been a high dropout rate and follow-up interviews suggested that logistical/scheduling issues played a large part in dropout rates, as did concern about the stigma of being part of an obesity treatment program.[13] A feasibility trial including an intervention group using a mobile health support system as an addition to standard care and a control group receiving standard care alone found that overall satisfaction, compliance, and dropout rate as well as BMI reductions were better in the intervention group.[14] Enhanced PREVENT is a study that tested 3 family-based telehealth interventions that were developed with input from a patient advisory council and pediatricians to target family concerns and encourage healthy lifestyle behavior. Three arms were created based on the feedback they received: healthy eating, physical activity, and a hybrid dyad. The hybrid dyad had the best compliance, but all telehealth interventions were well received with positive BMI outcomes.[15]

Overall, telehealth-based programs can be successful in treating pediatric obesity in rural settings. Dropout rates and compliance, however, continue to be barriers to effective treatment, which is the case in most pediatric obesity treatment centers, irrespective of whether the visits are in person or via telehealth. Little to no data exist to guide providers on which of the many programs available would be most efficacious for a particular environment. This decision needs to be made by the treating provider, considering the patient population, its needs, and area-specific treatment barriers, until more research is conducted and published.

Despite the expansion of more effective therapeutic options to treat obesity in children over the last 5 years, and positive outcomes for adolescent metabolic and bariatric surgery (MBS) as well as anti-obesity medications (AOM), there remain many barriers for patients and health care providers in being able to deliver these treatments equitably. The barriers can be considered across multiple sectors, from health care policy, attitudes, and bias to pediatric inclusion in research trials to best inform care (**Table 1**). Key barriers include access to treatment centers for those living in rural areas due to a lack of pediatric obesity medicine providers within reasonable driving distance from the patient's residence or due to a lack of transportation to get to the provider's office. Telehealth visits with pediatric obesity medicine specialists are an effective way to overcome this barrier, but challenges still exist, including a lack of access to adequate broadband to be able to successfully have a telehealth visit, as well as lack of insurance reimbursement for telehealth visits. The Federal Communications Commission 2018 outlines that more than 35% of US rural households were without broadband, and roughly 30 million had limited access. Other potential solutions involve using community properties, such as the town school or community hall, to conduct both in-person and telehealth visits.[16–18]

Table 1
Barriers to implementing care for pediatric patients with obesity in rural settings

Key Barriers	Concerns and Gaps	Opportunities
Access	Limited interdisciplinary obesity medicine centers in rural settings	Providing services via multiple modalities: telemedicine, satellite clinics, e-consults Support of policy to maintain and expand telehealth, reimbursement parity, support of health care systems to consider value-based care strategies to provide care to children living with obesity in rural areas
Insurance Coverage	Limited coverage for anti-obesity medications With advances in available effective treatments (behavioral, pharmacotherapy, surgery), there remains lack of coverage with <1% of patients with severe childhood obesity obtaining these therapies Current payment model impacts sustainability for both in-person and telemedicine care	Continued advocacy for State Medicaid coverage for anti-obesity medications Support of clinical team to assist with prior authorizations and appeal processes given current exclusion of these therapies Leveraging value-based care to support all patients and providers in the delivery of pediatric rural obesity care
Obesity Medical Education	Limited curriculum across interdisciplinary medical providers	Providing ECHO learning opportunities, building obesity medicine into formal curriculum for medical students, nursing, OT, PT, PhD, SW, physical education The growth of pediatric obesity medicine fellowships
Advocacy to Address Bias and Stigma	Data outline ongoing bias and stigma Greatly impacted by lack of understanding of the biologic basis for the pathophysiology of obesity Data highlighting persistence in negative stereotypes and stigmatization of patients with obesity by health care systems/providers	Support of patients and initiative to reduce obesity bias and stigma in the health care setting Support for existing efforts to educate policymakers and the public
Need for More Large-scale Pediatric Research and Clinical Trials	Required to better inform medical care as well as positively impact insurance coverage as often related to FDA approval, yet often with many years delay	Requires funding support to launch pediatric trials, creation of an obesity pediatric task force advocating for this research

While there has been an increase in providers obtaining board certification in obesity medicine, there continues to be a need for those in rural areas to obtain this specialty certification and to comfortably implement the recommended treatments. This includes having the resources needed to provide appropriate lifestyle modification guidance, prescribe pharmacotherapy, and when needed, refer to MBS. Providers need to be educated on the presence and content of the pediatric obesity guideline and to develop confidence in having conversations with patients about obesity treatment in ways that promote patient trust. Providers outside populated areas are less likely to have access to IHLBT or to be close to a center with specialty obesity care to provide MBS to adolescent patients. For these reasons, health systems need to embrace the provision of remote learning opportunities, such as Project Extension for Community Healthcare Outcomes (ECHO), E-consultations, and electronic health record support tools for providers. Providers and health systems need to advocate for better coverage for effective IHLBT programs, AOM, and MBS. Obesity treatment also can be hindered by the absence of needed ancillary providers in the treatment team, including dietitians, physical activity specialists, and behavioral health clinicians.

Issues with insurance coverage for aspects of pediatric obesity care are not confined to telehealth; several insurances, both public and private, do not provide reimbursement for dietitian visits, AOM, or MBS. Continuing advocacy for the appropriate reimbursement for the treatment of obesity is critical. This can be done at the insurance, local, state, and national level. Advocacy also involves the support of clinical research on pediatric obesity treatment options, for new modalities to be developed, studied, and for best practices to be updated.

Pre-pandemic, telemedicine to provide interdisciplinary pediatric obesity care was provided in a rural setting, which allowed collaboration with local primary care teams and increased access for patients. The experience provided a full spectrum of care with medical, dietary, behavioral health, and the use of AOM in a hybrid model.[19] The growth and expansion of telehealth since the COVID-19 pandemic have provided a valuable tool to providing obesity care. Leveraged lessons learned from telemedicine provide a vital path to bringing the best evidenced-based obesity specialty care to patients living in underserved, rural settings. Data support that most patients and providers have adopted the use of telemedicine as a standard of care modality. Additional benefits of telemedicine include improved insights into the patient's home environment, the ability to include more caregivers involved in the patient's care (grandparents, case workers, behavioral health provider), use of remote patient monitoring to obtain important anthropometric data, as well as less anxiety during visits for some patients with special health care needs, particularly those with anxiety, autism, and who have experienced obesity bias in prior health care settings. As we consider the impact and utility of telemedicine for providing best care for patients living in rural settings, applying the Reach, Effectiveness, Adoption, Implementation, Maintenance framework provides a structure for evaluating health interventions. Reviewing current challenges and opportunities for addressing pediatric obesity through this lens can create paths forward to improving care for children with obesity.

To ensure ongoing access via telemedicine, implementation strategies should be continually evaluated to consider settings, patient demographics, and geographic needs, along with revenue models to best meet these needs. Flattum and colleagues[4] outlined that a program design that may work in an urban setting may not translate directly to rural communities. Bailey and colleagues[20] highlight multiple strategies to consider when creating implementation and maintenance strategies. Both emphasized the importance of community partnerships and direct feedback from local health care providers and systems, and the importance of patients in the planning and implementation phases. Crawford and colleagues outlined a guide, the Digital Health Equity Framework, to assist in providing services, considering the risk of worsening existing disparities when using telehealth. These strategies can help inform policy and funding to support a multipronged approach to help address the challenges that are unique to providing care to pediatric patients with obesity, regardless of where they live.

For those patients living in rural settings, as has been our experience in Maine, the need to more creatively utilize all available modalities to ensure equitable access to care is vital. Our strategy, in Maine, has utilized the recommended multimodal approach. We have increased our obesity treatment specialty pediatric program size to eliminate our patient waiting list, created an e-consultation program for providers in the largest health system, expanded a telehealth obesity treatment program, and are working toward more robust satellite clinic options (**Figs. 1** and **2**). Funding for obesity treatment in our health system is buffered by a shared medical and surgical,

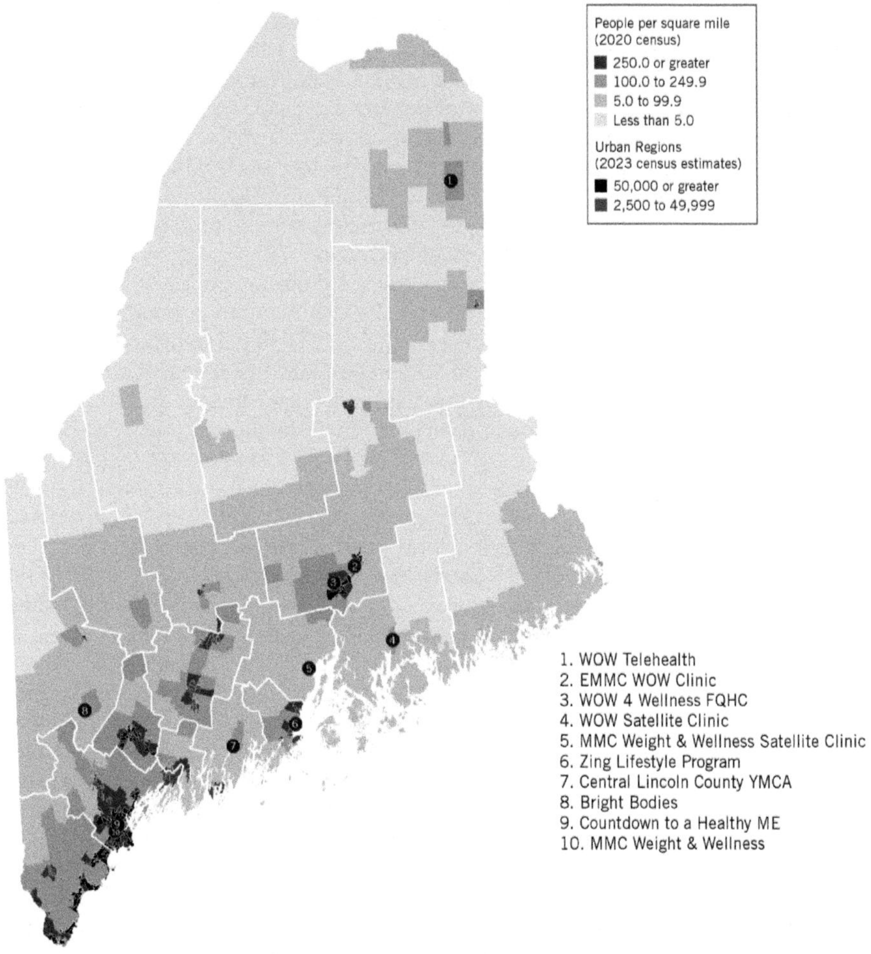

Fig. 1. Map of the state of Maine with location of pediatric weight management programs. Shaded areas indicate population density of various regions. (*Courtesy* Kate Allerding.)

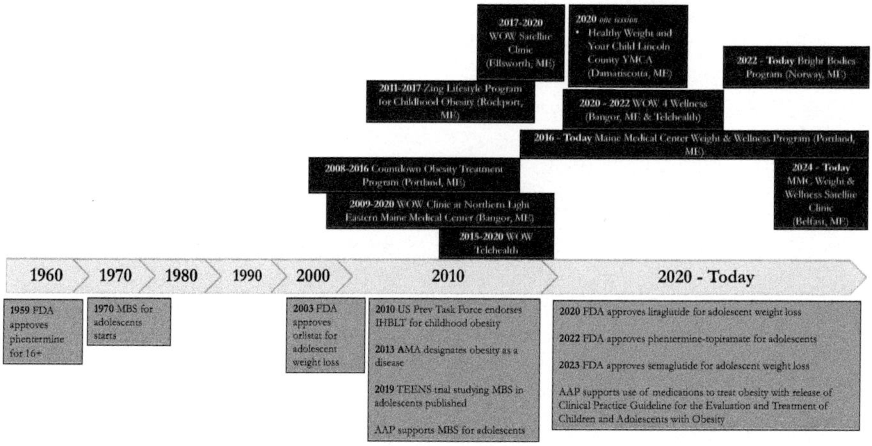

Fig. 2. Timeline of national pediatric obesity treatment milestones (*dark blue*) and pediatric weight management programs in the state of Maine (*maroon*). (*Courtesy* Meg Nadeau.)

adult and pediatric care model. We have delivered education on the CPG and effectiveness of MBS around the state at hospital and society-sponsored conferences and will soon be offering our second Project ECHO education on treatment of obesity. We have created a build in our electronic health record to guide obesity treatment decision-making and are working to implement IHBLT program options for patients. Despite the multipronged approach, we have been hindered by limited coverage of medications that are the Food and Drug Administration approved to treat children who have obesity, adding not only to the barriers of specialty care, but also to implementation of the CPG recommendations in primary care settings.

SUMMARY

The need for effective treatment of pediatric obesity is critical, as the disease's prevalence grows. Evaluation and treatment modalities are challenged by many factors, with rural and underserved populations most affected. The updated guidelines on pediatric obesity support the consideration of more aggressive forms of treatment to reduce the prevalence of the disease and its associated comorbidities. The implementation of these treatments in rural settings has improved with telehealth, but challenges still exist. Further research into techniques to expand and enhance pediatric obesity care in rural settings is needed; support of such research, as well as support of treatment options for patients by health care systems and third-party payors, is critical to achieving a reduction in the prevalence of pediatric obesity and its comorbidities.

DISCLOSURE

R. Conroy: none; C. Gordon: none; V. O'Hara: Speaker for Novo Nordisk.

REFERENCES

1. Hu K, Staiano AE. Trends in obesity prevalence among children and adolescents aged 2 to 19 years in the US From 2011 to 2020. JAMA Pediatr 2022;176(10):1037–9.

2. Cunningham SA, Hardy ST, Jones R, et al. Changes in the incidence of childhood obesity. Pediatrics 2022;150(2). e2021053708.
3. Ogden CL, Fryar CD, Hales CM, et al. Differences in obesity prevalence by demographics and urbanization in US children and adolescents, 2013-2016. JAMA 2018;319(23):2410–8.
4. Flattum C, Friend S, Horning M, et al. Family-focused obesity prevention program implementation in urban versus rural communities: a case study. BMC Publ Health 2021;21(1):1915.
5. McDaniel CE, Hall M, Berry JG. Trends in distance traveled for common pediatric conditions for rural-residing children. JAMA Pediatr 2024;178(1):80–1.
6. Hampl SE, Hassink SG, Skinner AC, et al. Clinical practice guideline for the evaluation and treatment of children and adolescents with obesity. Pediatrics 2023; 151(2). e2022060640.
7. Westfall JM, Mold J, Fagnan L. Practice-based research–"Blue Highways" on the NIH roadmap. JAMA 2007;297(4):403–6.
8. Balas EA, Boren SA. Managing clinical knowledge for health care improvement. Yearb Med Inform 2000;1:65–70.
9. Fischer F, Lange K, Klose K, et al. Barriers and strategies in guideline implementation—a scoping review. Healthcare 2016;4(3):3.
10. Janicke DM, Lim CS, Perri MG, et al. Featured article: behavior interventions addressing obesity in rural settings: the E-FLIP for kids trial. J Pediatr Psychol 2019; 44(8):889–901.
11. Hosseini H, Yilmaz A. Using telehealth to address pediatric obesity in rural Pennsylvania. Hosp Top 2019;97(3):107–18.
12. Nguyen L, Phan TL, Falini L, et al. Rural family satisfaction with telehealth delivery of an intervention for pediatric obesity and associated family characteristics. Child Obes 2023;20(3):147–54.
13. Hoft G, Forseth B, Trofimoff A, et al. Barriers to participation in a telemedicine-based, family-based behavioral group treatment program for pediatric obesity: qualitative findings from rural caregivers. Child Health Care 2024;53(1):60–75.
14. Johansson L, Hagman E, Danielsson P. A novel interactive mobile health support system for pediatric obesity treatment: a randomized controlled feasibility trial. BMC Pediatr 2020;20(1):447.
15. Poulsen MN, Hosterman JF, Wood GC, et al. Family-based telehealth initiative to improve nutrition and physical activity for children with obesity and its utility during COVID-19: a mixed methods evaluation. Front Nutr 2022;9:932514.
16. Novick MB, Wilson CT, Walker-Harding LR. Potential solutions for pediatric weight loss programs in the treatment of obesity in rural communities. Transl Behav Med 2019;9(3):460–7.
17. Cueto V, Sanders LM. Telehealth opportunities and challenges for managing pediatric obesity. Pediatr Clin North Am 2020;67(4):647–54.
18. DeSilva S, Vaidya SS. The application of telemedicine to pediatric obesity: lessons from the past decade. Telemed J e Health 2021;27(2):159–66.
19. O'Hara VM, Johnston SV, Browne NT. The paediatric weight management office visit via telemedicine: pre- to post-COVID-19 pandemic. Pediatr Obes 2020; 15(8):e12694.
20. Bailey JE, Gurgol C, Pan E, et al. Early patient-centered outcomes research experience with the use of telehealth to address disparities: scoping review. J Med Internet Res 2021;23(12):e28503.

Challenges and Opportunities of Pediatric Mental Health Practice in Rural America

Kari R. Harris, MD, FAAP[a,*],
Rachel M.A. Brown, MBBS, MRCPsych, FACPsych[b]

KEYWORDS

- Rural mental health care • Pediatric primary care clinicians
- Child and adolescent psychiatry • PMHCA • CPAP • FQHC • CCBHC
- Mental health crisis

KEY POINTS

- Rural youth are more likely struggle with mental illness, less likely to receive mental health care, and more likely to die by suicide than their urban peers.
- The United States currently has fewer than one-fifth of the needed child and adolescent psychiatrists to care for youth with severe psychiatric needs.
- Psychiatrists, psychologists, social workers, and therapists are needed to work alongside PCPs to carry out evidence-based mental health care for rural youth and families.

INTRODUCTION

Most of the United States has been deemed "rural" by the Health Resources and Services Administration (HRSA).[1] While a firm definition of "rural" does not exist, HRSA utilizes guidance from the US Census and the Office of Management and Budget making a functional description of rural to include any non-metropolitan and non-urban areas (or less than the defined threshold of 50,000 persons).[2] This definition identifies 15% to 19% of the population and 72% to 97% of the land as rural. Twenty-two percent of youth under age 18 live in rural areas.[2,3] Coupled with inadequate health care provision, much of the United States is underserved (**Fig. 1**)[4] with access to mental health care for children and adolescents (youth) being especially problematic.[5]

[a] Department of Pediatrics, University of Kansas School of Medicine - Wichita, 3243 East Murdock, Suite 402, Wichita, KS 67208, USA; [b] Psychiatry and Behavioral Sciences, University of Kansas School of Medicine-Wichita, 1010 North Kansas, Wichita, KS 67214, USA
* Corresponding author. 3243 East Murdock, Suite 402, Wichita, KS 67208.
E-mail address: kharris2@kumc.edu

Pediatr Clin N Am 72 (2025) 19–36
https://doi.org/10.1016/j.pcl.2024.07.025 pediatric.theclinics.com

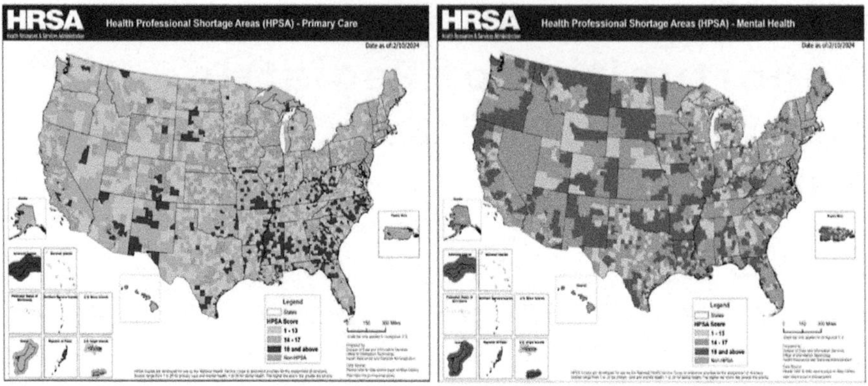

Fig. 1. Health professional shortage areas in the United States for primary care and mental health. (*Data from* Health Professional Shortage Areas (HSPA) - Primary Care. HRSA Data Warehouse. https://data.hrsa.gov/ExportedMaps/MapGallery/MUA.pdf.)

The American Academy of Child and Adolescent Psychiatrists (AACAP) estimates at least 47 Child and Adolescent Psychiatrists (CAPs) are needed per 100,000 youth under age 18. Only New York, Maine, Vermont, Massachusetts, and Hawaii meet this threshold, with the remaining 45 states and Puerto Rico having a "severe shortage."[6] The Substance Abuse and Mental Health Services Administration estimates 57,497 CAPs are needed to care for just the youth who meet criteria for severe emotional disturbances (SED). Currently, there are less than 10,000 CAPs in the country.[7] Unfortunately, the shortage is not only for CAPs; even more stark gaps have been identified for psychologists, social workers, non-physician prescribers, and other support professionals.[7]

SCOPE OF THE PROBLEM

Youth today are struggling with mental illness at unprecedented rates. Emergency departments, primary care clinics, and schools are seeing more youth with mental and behavioral health concerns than they have resources to support.[8–10] Primary care professionals (PCPs) feel out of their depth in diagnosing and managing youth with mental illness and lack specialists to whom youth can be referred.[11–13]

This crisis has been recognized by the American Academy of Pediatrics (AAP), the AACAP, the Children's Hospital Association, and the American Academy of Family Physicians.[14,15] Although the need permeates all geographic sites within North America, the hardship is especially prominent in Rural America. Not only are rural youth more likely to struggle with mental illness than their urban peers, but they are also more likely to have parents who struggle financially, have poorer mental health themselves, and have lower education levels than those living in urban communities.[9,16,17] Added to a backdrop of limited access to health care, these disparities can become a matter of life or death.[9,13,18] Adolescents in rural communities are more likely to die by suicide and fewer than half of adolescents with a mental health disorder receive treatment. Rural youth are less likely than urban youth to have access to appropriate mental health care, especially doctoral-level health professionals.[9,19]

There is a dearth of CAPs nationwide, with 70% of counties in the nation lacking a CAP (**Fig. 2**).[6] All mental health professionals, including CAPs, are more likely to practice in higher income and metropolitan counties, where residents also have higher levels of post-secondary education. In fact, the rural states of Indiana, Idaho, Kansas,

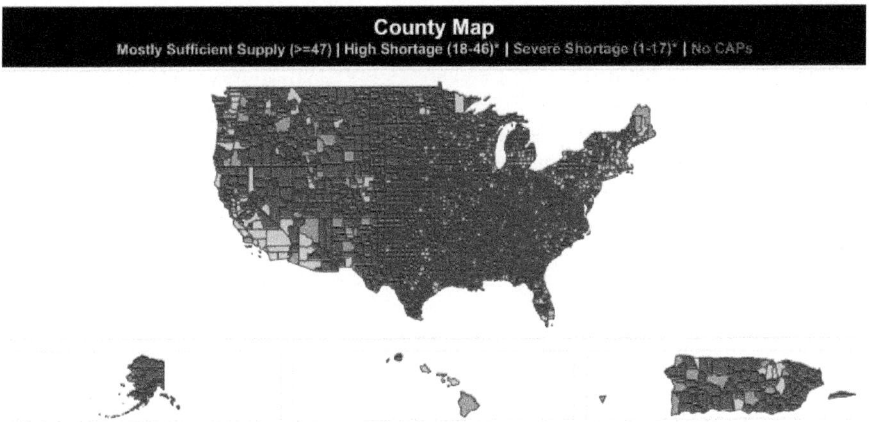

Fig. 2. Child and adolescent psychiatrist supply in the United States, 2022. (*Data from* AACAP. Practicing Child and Adolescent Psychiatrists. Workforce maps by State. Accessed February 2, 2024. https://www.aacap.org/aacap/Advocacy/Federal_and_State_Initiatives/Workforce_Maps/Home.aspx.)

North Dakota, South Carolina, and South Dakota saw a decline in the ratio of CAPs to youth between 2007 and 2016.[13]

As noted earlier, the United States currently has fewer than one-fifth of the needed CAPs to care for the youth with severe psychiatric needs. In the rural state of Kansas, 400 CAPs are needed to care for youth with SEDs, yet only 70 CAPs are practicing; only 10 practice outside the most urban area of the state (Northeast metro areas) (**Fig. 3**).[6]

The discrepancy in supply and demand for specialist pediatric mental health care expertise obligates PCPs to address mental health concerns from their patients.

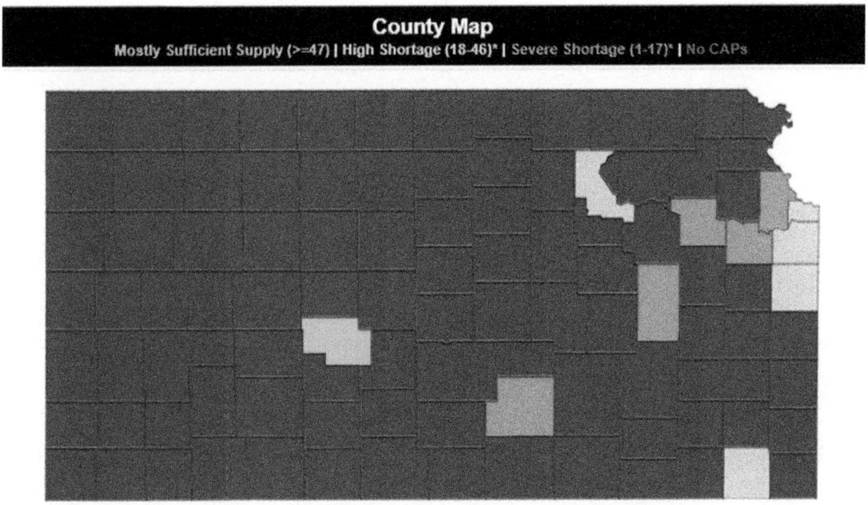

Fig. 3. Child and adolescent psychiatrist workforce in Kansas, 2022. (*Data from* AACAP. Practicing Child and Adolescent Psychiatrists. Workforce maps by State. Accessed February 2, 2024. https://www.aacap.org/aacap/Advocacy/Federal_and_State_Initiatives/Workforce_Maps/Home.aspx.)

Approximately 25% of pediatric health visits include a mental health complaint.[20] This is likely an underestimate of the need given that 42% of high school students endorse feelings of sadness or hopelessness and 1 in 10 have attempted suicide in the past year.[21] While many PCPs would prefer to refer youth out for mental health management, the lack of available specialists negates this preference and leaves PCPs with the choice of managing patients themselves or making referrals despite exceptional wait times.[22] Wait times to see specialists can be upward of 12 months, an unacceptable amount of time to wait to access potentially life-saving care.[23,24]

Like the workforce gap in mental health care access, rural states face shortages in primary care access (see **Fig. 2**).[4] The shortage in general pediatricians is especially pronounced in the rural state of Idaho where there are only 35 pediatricians per 100,000 youth.[25–27] While some states have up to 80 pediatricians per 100,000 youth, states that lack sufficient expertise in pediatric care suffer. Many rural communities rely on non-physician-level health care professionals to provide health care both in primary care and emergency settings. For instance, in Nebraska, very few counties have a pediatric primary care physician (**Fig. 4**)[28] and overall numbers of physicians in practice have been steadily declining. As of 2021, only 1675 physicians were practicing pediatrics in Nebraska as compared to 1087 physicians' assistants and 2048 advanced practice registered nurses.

According to Medicaid data in a mid-Atlantic state, prescribing by physicians (both psychiatrists and non-psychiatrists) decreased between 2012 and 2014 while a 50% increase was seen in prescribing of psychotropic medications by nurse practitioners.[29] Additionally, while psychiatrists and psychiatric nurse practitioners accounted for the majority (61.9%) of psychotropic prescriptions, over one-third (38.1%) of prescriptions were by non-specialists.[29] This is concerning, as research shows the use of antipsychotic medications in youth has risen dramatically. Specifically, within preschool-aged children there has been a 2-fold to 5-fold rise in antipsychotic prescribing.[30] This increase is occurring despite lack of evidence, known risk of harm, and lack of Food and Drug Administration approval for use in this age group.[30,31] Of further concern is that rural youth are more likely to receive

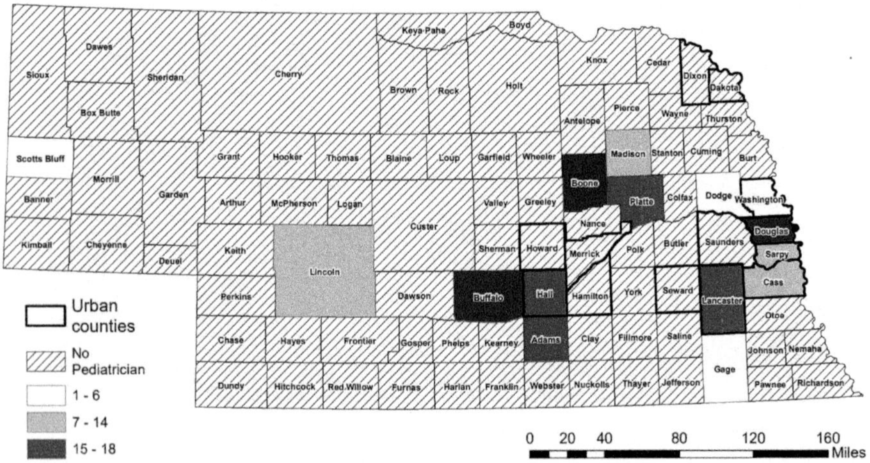

Fig. 4. Number of pediatric primary care physicians per 100, 000 youth in Nebraska, 2021. (*Data from* University of Nebraska Medical Center.[28])

psychopharmacotherapy for mental illness than counseling[9] despite evidence showing treatment with medication and counseling is superior to medication alone in many disorders in youth.[32,33]

Increased psychotropic prescriptions by non-specialists, highlights both the increase in mental health concerns in youth and the limited access to specialist care. Although multiple professional organizations have called pediatric clinicians to action to address the current mental health crisis,[15,34–36] pediatric clinicians throughout North America feel ill-equipped to treat mental illness in youth.[37–39] This is not surprising given the lack of training in pediatric mental health received by PCPs. Canadian pediatric PCPs view pediatric mental health care as a highly specialized area of medicine and cite many barriers to providing this care.[40] In fact, specialists do receive far more training in psychiatry than PCPs. A physician specialized in general psychiatry completes roughly 200 hours of supervised clinical time each month of a 4-year residency totaling nearly 10,000 hours over the course of specialization; CAPs then have an additional 2 years of pediatric-specific psychiatry training.[41–43] While studies quantifying the actual hours of psychiatric training for pediatric clinicians are sorely lacking, we know for PCPs, the number of training hours drastically decreases. According to the Accreditation Council for Graduate Medical Education, pediatricians are required to have 4 weeks each in 2 mental health-heavy rotations: developmental and behavioral pediatrics, and adolescent medicine; and beginning in 2025, an additional 4 weeks of mental health will be required. Other than these standardized rotations, pediatric and family medicine residents manage mental illness during continuity clinics and specialty rotations and can choose from mental health-related electives, including child and adolescent psychiatry where they are precepted by the most specialized experts in child mental illness.[42] Physicians also receive some training in mental health during undergraduate medical training although this is also not well quantified and may range from 0 to 130 hours depending on the medical school attended.[44] Comparatively, nurse practitioners specializing in psychiatric care are required to have 500 hours of supervised clinical time in psychiatry over a 5-year period, although this time is not necessarily specific to *youth* with psychiatric illnesses.[41] Additional Pediatric Primary Care Mental Health Specialty certification can be sought by nurse practitioners and requires between 1000 and 2000 post-graduate hours over 5 years, but preceptor supervision is not required[45] bringing into question the fidelity to evidence-based medicine and quality of care. Physician assistants and general nurse practitioners receive the least amount of pediatric mental health training and while literature quantifying this training is even more scant, interviews reveal that in some programs no in-depth pediatric mental health training occurs (Harris K.R., MD, Interview scripts unpublished data 2024).

There have been efforts to remedy this lack of education in training. The AAP published "Mental Health Competencies for Pediatric Practice" in 2019 as a revision to their 2009 policy statement. This affirms the important role pediatricians have in preventing, identifying, and managing mental illness.[46] Additionally, the AAP has a 2-part guideline to assist pediatric clinicians in the management of adolescent depression in primary care.[34,35] Unfortunately, these recommendations are less than a decade old and there is a known practice gap of 16 to 17 years for new recommendations to reach clinical practice.[47] Simultaneously, the rate of emergency room visits for mental health disorders has been increasing.[48] The federal government has adopted policy and provided funding to support pediatric clinicians both in practice and in training, as well as grow the workforce in multiple disciplines required for high-level pediatric mental health care.[49–52]

CURRENT INTERVENTIONS

Telehealth

Telehealth alleviates many barriers to accessing mental health care, especially for rural patients. Since the coronavirus disease 2019 pandemic, the use of telehealth has greatly expanded. Emergency orders both kept people at home and expanded the allowances for telehealth. New policies addressed historical barriers clinicians faced including low reimbursement rates for televisits, which were increased during and upheld following the pandemic. Telehealth allowed rural patients to seek care from the comfort of home rather than traveling to a distant clinic.[53,54] Telehealth access may have also helped decrease stigma around mental health care, a challenge that occurs more in rural communities than urban ones. This is partly due to the unique challenges of providing mental health care in rural communities. Social and professional challenges exist for patients and clinicians as both likely work, live, and interact with each other outside of their patient-professional relationship.[55] Receiving care virtually from a professional outside of the local community may help alleviate some of these unique challenges of providing and receiving mental health care in smaller, rural communities.

Albeit helpful in some ways, telehealth far from addresses all access barriers. Lab work is unavailable virtually and lack of in-person visits can hinder rapport between clinician and patient. Telehealth has been described as an "intermediate" step to health care: helpful for preliminary screening and follow-up but not appropriate for all care.[53] Further, while telehealth can address maldistribution of mental health specialists, the overall issue of workforce shortage remains unsolved. If a psychiatrist in an urban town blocks time to care for rural youth virtually, they sacrifice time seeing youth in-person. So, while this may help in other fields of medicine where there is a sufficient supply of professionals, it does not help the overall workforce crisis in pediatric mental health. Still, the increased availability of telehealth care has been a welcomed change in service provision allowing youth to miss less school for travel to specialists and keeping adults more productive in rural communities. Telehealth has also been utilized to offer consultations to pediatric clinicians to both educate on mental health care and extend management (**Box 1**).[56] Programs like Pediatric Mental Health Care Access (PMHCA) Programs or Child Psychiatry Access Programs (CPAP) utilize telehealth for direct consultations with psychiatrists and as a learning tool for pediatric clinicians to build expertise and comfort in pediatric mental health care.[10,57]

Box 1
Colorado case example

In an innovative program in rural Colorado, child and adolescent psychiatrists work as part of an integrated care team to provide interprofessional mental health care to pediatric patients. The model includes masters-level behavioral health clinicians (BHC), pediatric primary care professionals (PCPs), psychologists, and a child and adolescent psychiatrist (CAP). The PCPs serve as team leads and manage all patient care and prescriptions but can request a consult from the CAP for care beyond their comfort level. The consult is then organized by the BHC. The BHC participates in the consult with the CAP, patient, and family and this direct care is followed by a wrap up session with the same team and including the psychologist and PCP. The PCP then carries out any management plans.

From (A multidisciplinary, team-based teleconsultation approach to enhance child mental health services in rural pediatrics)[56]; with permission.

Pediatric Mental Health Access Programs/Child Psychiatry Access Programs

Funded through HRSA beginning in 2018, 54 PMHCA programs now exist across the United States (**Fig. 5**).[50] Based on the original CPAP in Massachusetts, the overarching goal of PMHCA programs is to "promote behavioral health integration into pediatric primary care by using telehealth modalities to provide high-quality and timely detection, assessment, treatment, and referral for children and adolescents, with behavioral health conditions, using evidence-based practices and methods."[58] Although this goal is integral to each program, each PMHCA has unique components (**Fig. 6**).

Most rely on CAPs and child psychologists to provide consultation to pediatric clinicians regarding management of mental illness. Data supporting uptake, satisfaction, and utilization by pediatric clinicians have been reported for PMHCA/CPAP programs and pediatric clinicians have reported a gain in skills, knowledge, comfort, and confidence following engagement in programs.[59–61]

North Dakota, a vastly rural and frontier state, hosts a PMHCA that provides peer-to-peer consultation between PCP and specialists. Care coordination for patients and families are also available through a PMHCA-partnering organization. The North Dakota program also offers ongoing trainings to pediatric clinicians through Project Extension for Community Healthcare Outcomes and annual symposiums.[62]

Mental Health Training Programs

Excellent primary care training is necessary for pediatric clinicians practicing in rural communities; however, historically, this has not included pediatric mental health care. To train PCPs in pediatric mental health care, psychiatric specialists are needed in rural communities. CAPs are the most highly trained experts in pediatric mental illness. As outlined earlier, training for these specialist physicians requires 4 years of undergraduate medical education, 3 to 4 years of general psychiatry residency training, and an additional 2 years of child and adolescent fellowship training. CAPs are trained in pathophysiological, psychopharmacological, and psychotherapeutic

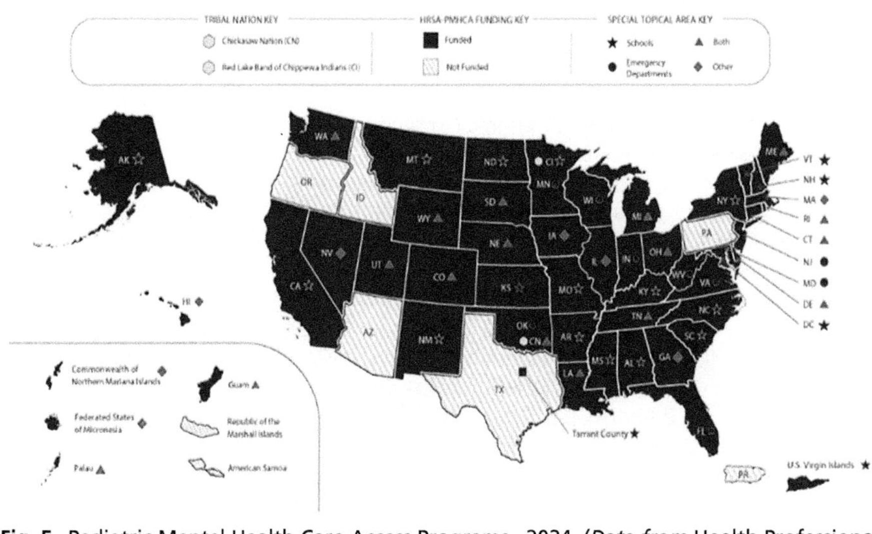

Fig. 5. Pediatric Mental Health Care Access Programs , 2024. (*Data from* Health Professional Shortage Areas (HSPA) - Mental Health. HRSA Data Warehouse. https://mchb.hrsa.gov/programs-impact/programs/pediatric-mental-health-care-access.[50])

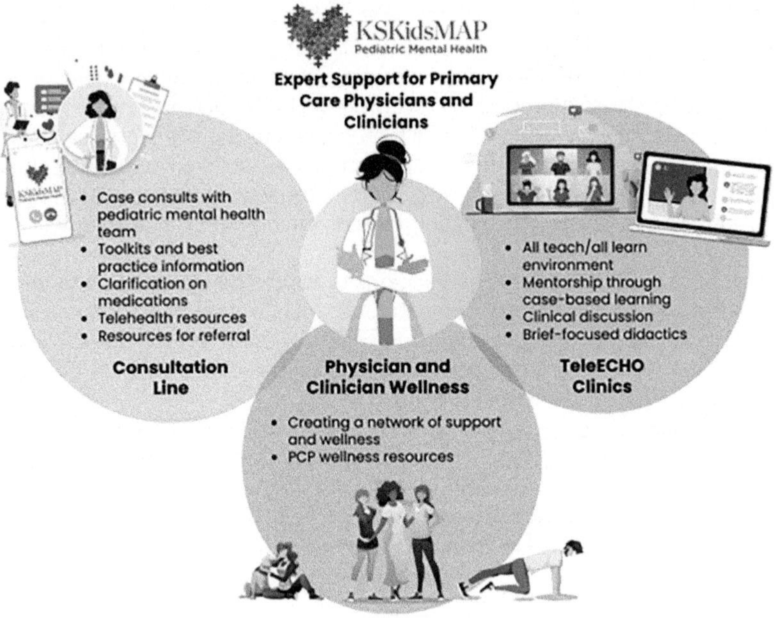

The Kansas PMHCA program, KSKidsMAP, has 3 main pillars: 1) A free consultation line that PCPs can call to receive pediatric mental health care advice from the expert pediatric mental health team of child and adolescent psychiatry, child psychology, social work, and pediatric primary care; 2) TeleECHO Clinic sessions held bi-monthly for case-based learning with the expert pediatric mental health team; and 3) PCP wellness resources to support PCPs experiencing emotional burdens when caring for youth with mental illness. The program was funded in 2019 and awarded continuation funding in 2023. New funding has allowed program expansion to include school-based health consultations and KSKidsMAP programming for Autism, neurodevelopmental disorders, and intellectual disabilities (KANDID).

Fig. 6. Kansas case example. (*From* the university of Kansas School of Medicine-Wichita; with permission.)

management of pediatric mental illness. No other health professional has this level of training in pediatric mental illness. This expertise makes them the most qualified to teach pediatric clinicians about mental health disorders. Regrettably, there are not enough CAPs to meet patient care needs, let alone teaching needs. It has become imperative, that pediatric clinicians become well-trained, knowledgeable, and comfortable managing less complex mental illness so that youth with more complex psychiatric needs can be seen by these specialists. Several new training programs have recently been funded through HRSA that aim to equip pediatric clinicians with these skills. Further, programs now exist to train CAPs and child psychologists with an emphasis on underserved and rural populations.

At least 2 current Primary Care Training and Enhancement (PCTE) programs funded by HRSA provide training to pediatric clinicians related to mental and behavioral health care. The purpose of the PCTE-Physician Assistant Rural Training in Behavioral Health program is to develop clinical rotations regarding behavioral health and substance use for physician assistant students in rural communities. The purpose of the PCTE-Residency Training in Mental and Behavioral Health (PCTE-RTMB) is to train primary care physician residents in mental, behavioral, and substance use care for pediatric, adolescent, young adult, and other at-risk or exposed populations. Both programs should help equip future rural pediatric clinicians with expertise to manage youth with mental health disorders.[63,64] A third HRSA program, Behavioral Health Workforce Education and Training (BHWET) Program for Professionals is working to increase and improve distribution of behavioral health professionals especially those focused on the care of youth and young adults.[49] The BHWET program becomes increasingly important as the need for these specialists increases both for patient care and for the education of other health professionals. These 3 HRSA programs overlap with the goals of the PMHCA programs and can integrate synergistically to achieve the common goal of improved mental and behavioral health care in rural communities (**Box 2**).

Rural Primary Care Training Programs

Programs that build up local health professionals in rural communities are important. These programs increase capacity of pediatric clinicians, extend the reach of pediatric mental health specialists, and allow care for patients by trusted, local clinicians. The latter point is especially relevant in rural communities. Rural parents have higher levels of concern receiving care from mental health professionals when compared with their urban counterparts. Given the extreme shortage of mental health professionals, many providing treatment to rural youth come from outside local communities. This can heighten distrust of the professional and hinder treatment.[9] Building up local pediatric clinicians through initiatives like PMHCA programs helps to address this barrier.

Building capacity of local, existing rural clinicians is only 1 piece of the puzzle. As previously stated, rural communities often lack even PCPs so supporting programs that train pediatric clinicians to serve rural communities is vital to addressing the mental health crisis. Undergraduate medical education curricula with a focus on rural

Box 2
Synergistic Programs

The KU School of Medicine-Wichita developed 3 Health Resources and Services Administration (HRSA)-funded projects to enhance the pediatric mental health care workforce. The first, Kansas Kids Mental Health Access Program (KSKidsMAP) Pediatric Mental Health Care Access (see Box 2) builds capacity of PCPs to manage pediatric mental illness. The second, "Addressing Youth Mental and Behavioral Health Illness in primary care (AYM HI)" Primary Care Training and Enhancement, enhances education for pediatric residents and faculty to address mental illnesses and substance use disorders. The third program, Kansas Educating Excellent Psychologists and Psychiatrists for Underserved/Rural Youth Patients (KEEP UP), a HRSA Behavioral Health Workforce Education and Training program, aims to sustainably increase the supply of highly trained psychiatrists and psychologists through comprehensive training in community settings. All 3 programs work synergistically to meet individual program objectives while achieving a common goal to increase access to quality pediatric mental health care. KSKidsMAP meets needs of all 3 programs through case-based learning during Tele Extension for Community Healthcare Outcomes (TeleECHO) Clinics and provides training and teaching opportunities to KEEP UP trainees. KEEP UP participants gain real life experience working with KSKidsMAP PCPs and serving as consulting experts and educators. KEEP UP benefits KSKidsMAP with increased availability of consultants and education from highly trained mental health professionals. AYM HI integrates seamlessly into these programs providing opportunities for KEEP UP trainees to teach pediatric residents, provide consultations, and interface with primary care and academic medicine settings. All 3 programs utilize and support our school-based health clinics, bringing the synergy of the programs into the community allowing for real-world application of learned skills.

From the University of Kansas School of Medicine-Wichita; with permission.

medicine can positively impact the rural health workforce. Many medical schools have programs promoting rural practice that consistently produce physicians who practice rurally. Fostering rural interest early is one strategy to build the rural pediatric workforce and data show these rural physicians remain in rural practice long term.[65]

Graduate Medical Education is the next step when training rural physicians. According to the American Medical Association's Residency and Fellowship database , 17/218 pediatric and 213/761 family medicine residency programs in the United States offer rural tracks.[66] Unfortunately, most family medicine residents (91%) receive no rural training. This is significant as residents who train even for short periods in rural settings are at least twice as likely to practice rurally.[67] Finally, residents are most likely to practice professionally where they train, and most residency programs are located in urban and suburban areas.[68,69] Those residency programs that do expose trainees to practice in Rural Health Clinics (RHC), Federally Qualified Health Centers (FQHC), or Critical Access Hospitals show higher rates of graduates who remain practicing in those locations even after 5 years.[65]

Federally Qualified Health Clinics and Rural Health Clinics

FQHCs illustrate another health care opportunity in rural communities. Both FQHCs and RHCs exist in rural communities and provide a majority of health care. FQHCs, established in 1991, expand the services RHCs offer to include comprehensive and preventive care services. FQHCs have seen a significant increase (83%) in overall mental and behavioral health visits since 2010 making them an important player in addressing mental illness in youth.[68] Often staffed by primary care physicians, nurse practitioners, and physicians' assistants, managing mental health within these clinics can be overwhelming and under-resourced. A 2023 report by the Bipartisan Policy Center acknowledged challenges in providing mental health care in these facilities and highlighted the need for training, resources, and reimbursement changes. The report, and subsequent policy recommendations, propose integrated care as a solution, citing evidence, cost-savings, and convenience as opportunities for integrated care, though it also addresses multiple challenges to integrating care in rural settings.[68] FQHCs and RHCs help to address the payment disparity for rural pediatric clinicians who rely extensively on Medicaid and are unable to cap their underinsured population for sheer lack of other access for these patients. Currently, in rural areas, 1 in 4 patients under 65 are enrolled in Medicaid. Medicaid pays roughly 30% less than Medicare, which pays 30% less than private payers. This is even more disparate when covering primary care and mental health services as compared to specialist services.[70] FQHCs and RHCs address this challenge by providing enhanced reimbursement rates for Medicaid and Medicare services. While beyond the scope of this article, payment reform and progress toward integrated care in rural communities seems to be a promising solution. FQHCs are key players in this reform.

Community Mental Health Centers and Certified Community Behavioral Health Clinics

Though more recently established, FQHCs have similarities with a much older model of care: community mental health. In the past 75 years, there has been a push for more community-based mental health care. Before this, most psychiatrically ill patients were managed at institutions with varying quality. When President John Kennedy signed the Community Mental Health Act in 1963, psychiatric institutions closed, funding was moved to states, and community mental health centers (CMHCs) began forming.[71] CMHCs receive federal funding from Medicaid and Medicare and follow specific guidelines. Patients must receive care from treatment teams that provide coordination of services.[72] However, levels and types of care have varied, and programming has not always been evidence-based, or even well-received by patients. This is partly due to differences in funding sources, funding levels, and available professionals to staff the clinics.[71,73] Additionally, CMHCs were limited to mental health care and FQHCs to primary medical care with very little communication between clinicians. This model effectively separated the "mind" from the "body." As more holistic care has become favorable, and due to workforce shortages and other aforementioned challenges, mental health care is more commonly becoming part of primary care. Unfortunately, PCPs report many barriers to referring to CMHCs including poor return communication, lack of evidence-based approaches, dissatisfaction of patients, and parent refusal for their child to receive CMHC services (Harris K, unpublished data, interviews with PCPs through Kansas Kids Mental Health Access Program). The US Department of Health and Human Services has recognized the shortcomings of the CMHC model and in 2017 began implementing a new model for community behavioral health care.

Established by the Protecting Access to Medicare Act of 2014, Certified Community Behavioral Health Clinics (CCBHCs) are a newer model of community mental health built on lessons learned from the CMHC model. Funding for this model is based on a Prospective Payment System providing an enhanced monthly Medicaid reimbursement at a fixed cost per qualifying service delivered. Rates are determined by expected costs of each clinic. This payment overhaul has allowed services to be covered at cost rather than at a loss and provided for more competitive pay rates for qualified staff. CCBHCs were piloted in 8 states beginning in 2017, with the aim to improve community behavioral health by making it more accessible and whole-person focused. CCBHCs are required to offer the following services: 24/7 crisis services; screening, assessment, diagnosis and risk assessment; treatment planning; outpatient mental health and substance use services; targeted case management; outpatient primary care; screening and monitoring; community-based mental health care for veterans; peer, family support and counselor services; psychiatric rehabilitation services.[73–75] All CCBHCs are required to have a psychiatrist serve in the role of medical director of the clinic. Given that CCBHCs serve youth with complex mental illnesses including SEDs, this level of expertise is necessary; although employing a psychiatric nurse practitioner to fill this role is allowable if a psychiatrist is unavailable. In the pilot, 91% of the programs employed a psychiatrist as medical director. Additional required CCBHCs staff includes a behavioral health care prescriber who can practice independently, credentialed substance use specialists, and professionals with expertise in trauma-informed care; though with continued workforce shortages recruiting and retaining staff has been an ongoing challenge.[75] Still, it seems the CCBHC model has been able to address many of the pitfalls of the older CMHC model and many states are adopting this practice (**Fig. 7**).

Incentives for Rural Health Professionals

One reason the CCHBC model has gained favor is the enhanced payment for mental health services. Historically, mental health care has been underpaid and consumed more time than typical primary care visits. In rural communities, where health professionals are scarce, recruitment is a constant and everchanging endeavor. Convincing a pediatric clinician to come to a small community to be underpaid and overworked is difficult. Incentivizing health professionals to work rurally has been a promising practice since at least 1972 when the National Health Service Corps (NHSC) began recruiting primary care physicians into rural communities; likewise, Title VII of the Public Health Service Act financially supports the training of primary care physicians.[65,76]

Oklahoma, with a rich population of Indigenous Americans, was one of the demonstration states for the new CCHBC model. Three clinics in 19 service locations were piloted initially and the program has now grown to reach all Oklahomans needing care. The state utilizes a dashboard for each unique patient to inform the treatment team on the services provided and level of coordination occurring. One parent is quoted on the state website illustrating the integrated care happening for her child and family:

"When I first brought [my daughter] to Systems of Care she was a withdrawn, anxious, and depressed child. With the help of SOC she has become a happier, outgoing kid who loves life, writing, singing, and art... I want to thank SOC for teaching not only her but our whole family coping skills and communication skills to deal with things in life as they come. I don't know where we would be if we didn't have SOC."

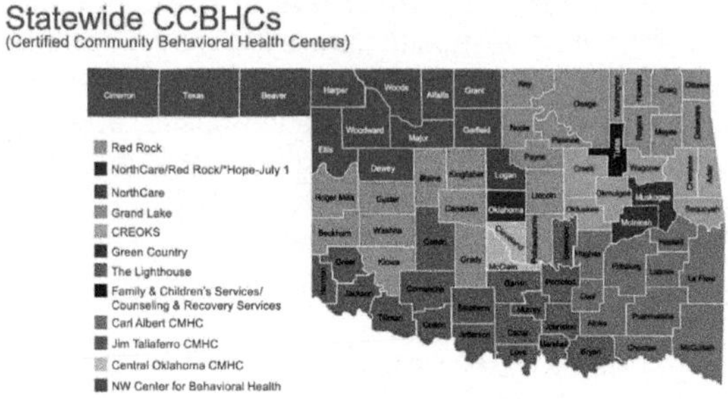

Fig. 7. Oklahoma's Certified Community Behavioral Health Clinic story. (*Data from* the Oklahoma Mental health and substance abuse; with permission.)

Several other federal programs have helped physicians with loan repayment, scholarships, financial bonuses, and waivers of an immigration requirement for non-US citizen physicians (State 30 J-1 Visa Waiver Programs)[76] (**Box 3**).[77] In 2017, federal and state-funded incentive programs were estimated to have assisted placement of 6500 physicians into rural and underserved areas.[76] Program requirements vary but all include a term of service in the underserved community. Similar rural recruitment programs also exist for physician assistants and nurse practitioners.

Unfortunately, anecdotal evidence suggests that incentivized professionals will often serve their contracted time and then relocate to more urbanized communities. This leaves communities without a health care professional or with frequent turnover, exacerbating the lack of trust for professionals in these communities. Limited research suggests incentives that offer loan repayment have improved retention for physicians in rural or underserved communities when compared to J-1 waiver programs.[78] A systematic review supported this showing NHSC scholarship physicians were likely to remain in rural practice 8 to 16 years after initial assignment.[65] Reasons for this are unclear and likely multimodal, though a theory suggests loan repayment programs incentivize physicians who would have worked in rural communities regardless of the incentive.[77] In fact, several studies have found growing up in rural areas is associated

Box 3
An innovative incentive in Rural Kansas

Recruiting full scope primary care physicians is a challenge in any rural community. The story was no different for Kearny County Hospital in Lakin, KS, population 2100. The critical access hospital provides full scope care for much of southwest Kansas. However, unlike many rural communities, diversity is plentiful with patients representing 22 different countries and a mission-minded board of directors. The hospital uses this to their advantage, recruiting from the family international medicine fellowship in Wichita, Kansas and offering paid leave of 8 weeks annually for these physicians to pursue mission work.

From the university of Kansas School of Medicine-Wichita[77]; with permission.

with rural physician practice,[65] again emphasizing the importance of fostering interest in rural practice early in medical training.

While PCPs are the cornerstone of pediatric care in rural communities, innovations are also needed to bring psychiatric specialists, psychologists, and therapists to rural areas. The Centers for Medicare and Medicaid Services offers financial bonuses to psychiatrists working in mental health professional shortage area but not to other health professionals—though expansion to other health professionals has been recommended by the Bipartisan Policy Center.[68] Psychiatrists, psychologists, social workers, and therapists are needed to work alongside PCPs to carry out evidence-based mental health care for rural youth and families.

SUMMARY

Practicing medicine in Rural America is rich with opportunities and wrought with challenges. Practicing pediatric mental health care in rural communities further exacerbates these unique challenges. On one hand, pediatric clinicians are well-placed to care for their patients struggling with mental health concerns. The opportunity to understand complex psychosocial contributors only is known from caring for parents, extended families, and living within the social context of the community can certainly aid clinicians in assessing and managing mental illness. On the other hand, knowledge, comfort, and experience in managing pediatric mental illness remain significant barriers to patients receiving high-quality, evidence-based care. Though still lacking overall, resources are available to support rural pediatric clinicians in this endeavor. Programs that aim to build up existing rural clinicians and educate and attract new health care professionals to rural areas are critical to addressing the pediatric mental health crisis. However, PCPs need the support of highly specialized CAPs both for this education and for consultation when they feel out of their depth. Therefore, initiatives aimed at increasing CAPs and child and adolescent psychologists are necessary. Pediatric patients have complex inner-workings of mind and body and are highly affected by their environments. Care for youth should be family-centered, holistic, and team-based. These goals are at the heart of the CCBHC and FQHC models. To be successful though, care must be financially sustainable for clinicians and systems. Further, programs that support clinicians and systems must remain adequately funded until the gap in pediatric mental health care access and quality is closed.

CLINICS CARE POINTS

- A National Emergency in Pediatric Mental Health has been declared by multiple child-serving medical organizations.
- Youth living in Rural America have increased rates of mental illness and inadequate resources to address this.
- Rural pediatric clinicians are well placed to care for youth in primary care practice but need support. This includes education, resources, and experts in pediatric mental illness with whom clinicians can consult and to whom they can refer youth with complex illness.
- Programs and systems are currently available to build capacity in pediatric clinicians to care for youth with mental illness and to recruit and support rural clinicians. Examples include Pediatric Mental Health Care Access Programs, incentive programs to recruit clinicians to rural areas, and enhanced Medicaid reimbursement for qualifying health centers.

- Additional funding for existing programs, new innovative programs, and training for child and adolescent psychiatrists are ongoing needs that will help address the pediatric mental health crisis in North America.

DISCLOSURE

Drs R.M. Anne Brown and K.R. Harris receive federal funding from Health Resources and Services Administration (HRSA), United States as key personnel of 3 grant awards: a PMHCA program (KSKidsMAP), a BWHET program (KEEP UP), and a PCTE-RTMB program (AYM HI).

REFERENCES

1. Critical access hospitals and Federal Office of Rural Health Policy (FORHP) Rural Health Areas. Map gallery. July 9, 2021. Accessed January 20, 2024.
2. Health Resources & Services Administration. Defining rural population. HRSA. 2024. Available at: https://www.hrsa.gov/rural-health/about-us/what-is-rural. Accessed February 10, 2024.
3. CNMP JB. Measuring America: our changing landscape. Census.gov; 2021. . Accessed January 20, 2024.
4. Medically underserved areas/populations. Map gallery. Available at: https://data.hrsa.gov/ExportedMaps/MapGallery/MUA.pdf. Accessed January 20, 2024.
5. Health Professional Shortage Areas (HPSA) - mental health. Map gallery. Available at: https://data.hrsa.gov/ExportedMaps/MapGallery/HPSAMH.pdf. Accessed January 20, 2024.
6. AACAP. Practicing Child and Adolescent Psychiatrists. Workforce maps by state. Available at: https://www.aacap.org/aacap/Advocacy/Federal_and_State_Initiatives/Workforce_Maps/Home.aspx. Accessed February 2, 2024.
7. Behavioral Health Workforce Report - Annapolis coalition. 2022. Available at: https://annapoliscoalition.org/wp-content/uploads/2021/03/behavioral-health-workforce-report-SAMHSA-2.pdf. Accessed January 20, 2024.
8. Radhakrishnan L, Leeb RT, Bitsko RH, et al. Pediatric Emergency Department Visits Associated with Mental Health Conditions Before and During the COVID-19 Pandemic — United States, January 2019–January 2022. MMWR Morb Mortal Wkly Rep 2022;71:319–24.
9. Blackstock Jacob KBC, Angela M, Mauk GW, et al. Achieving access to mental health care for school-aged children in rural communities. Rural Educat 2018; 39(1):15.
10. Harris K, Aguila Gonzalez A, Vuong N, et al. Understanding pediatric mental health in primary care: needs in a rural state. Clin Pediatr 2018;62(5):441–8.
11. Bettencourt AF, Ferro RA, Williams J-LL, et al. Pediatric primary care provider comfort with mental health practices: A needs assessment of regions with shortages of treatment access. Acad Psychiatr 2021;45(4):429–34.
12. Steele M, Zayed R, Davidson B, et al. Referral patterns and training needs in psychiatry among Primary Care Physicians in Canadian Rural/Remote Areas. J Can Acad Child Adolesc Psychiatry 2012;21(2):111–23. PMID: 22548108; PMCID: PMC3338177.
13. McBain RK, Kofner A, Stein BD, et al. Growth and distribution of child psychiatrists in the United States: 2007–2016. Am J Pediatr 2019;144(6).
14. Family physicians urge policymakers to focus on mental health care for children families. AAFP. 2021. Available at: https://www.aafp.org/news/media-center/statements/

family-physicians-mental-health-care-children-families.html. Accessed February 10, 2024.

15. Aap-AACAP-Cha Declaration of a national emergency in Child and Adolescent Mental Health. 2021. Available at: https://www.aap.org/en/advocacy/child-and-adolescent-healthy-mental-development/aap-aacap-cha-declaration-of-a-national-emergency-in-child-and-adolescent-mental-health/. Accessed January 30, 2024.
16. Morales DA, Barksdale CL, Beckel-Mitchener AC. A call to action to address rural mental health disparities. J Transl Sci 2020;4(5):463–7. Available at: https://www.cambridge.org/core/journals/journal-of-clinical-and-translational-science/article/call-to-action-to-address-rural-mental-health-disparities/FF7E3D53F66B2BA0DE572BC2B30B10CE. Accessed February 8, 2024.
17. Working together, we can help children in rural communities thrive. Centers for Disease Control and Prevention. 2023. Available at: https://www.cdc.gov/childrensmentalhealth/features/rural-health.html. Accessed February 8, 2024.
18. Fehr KK, Leraas BC, Littles MMD. Behavioral health needs, barriers, and parent preferences in rural pediatric primary care. J Pediatr Psychol 2020;45(8):910–20.
19. Hastings SL, Cohn TJ. Challenges and opportunities associated with rural mental health practice. Rural Ment Health 2013;37(1):37–49.
20. Poynter SE, McNeal-Trice K, Gonzalez del Rey J. Addressing the behavioral and mental health educational gap in pediatric residency training. Am J Pediatr 2020;146(1).
21. High school YRBS. Centers for Disease Control and Prevention. Available at: https://nccd.cdc.gov/Youthonline/App/Results.aspx?TT=A&OUT=0&SID=HS&QID=QQ&LID=XX&YID=2021&LID2=&YID2=&COL=S&ROW1=N&ROW2=N&HT=QQ&LCT=LL&FS=S1&FR=R1&FG=G1&FA=A1&FI=I1&FP=P1&FSL=S1&FRL=R1&FGL=G1&FAL=A1&FIL=I1&FPL=P1&PV=&TST=False&C1=&C2=&QP=G&DP=1&VA=CI&CS=Y&SYID=&EYID=&SC=DEFAULT&SO=ASC. Accessed January 20, 2024.
22. Pignatiello A, Stasiulis E, Solimine C, et al. Lessons learned in a physician referral to pediatric telemental health services program. J Can Acad Child Adolesc Psychiatry 2019;28(3):99–104.
23. Sullivan K, George P, Horowitz K. Addressing national workforce shortage by funding child psychiatry access programs. Pediatrics 2021;147(1):e20194012.
24. Steinman KJ, Shoben AB, Dembe AE, et al. How long do adolescents wait for psychiatry appointments? Community ment. Health J 2015;52(7):782–9.
25. General pediatricians U.S. state and county maps. General Pediatricians U.S. State and County Maps | The American Board of Pediatrics. 2023. Available at: https://www.abp.org/dashboards/general-pediatricians-us-state-and-county-maps. Accessed January 20, 2024.
26. Dutton A. Idaho has about 40 pediatricians for every 100,000 kids. A new venture could help. Idaho Capital Sun; 2022. Available at: https://idahocapitalsun.com/2022/02/07/idaho-has-about-40-pediatricians-for-every-100000-kids-a-new-venture-could-help/. Accessed January 7, 2024.
27. WSJ News Exclusive. Children are dying in ill-prepared emergency rooms across America. Wall St J 2023. Available at: https://www.wsj.com/health/healthcare/hospitals-emergency-rooms-cost-childrens-lives-d6c9fc23. Accessed February 14, 2024.
28. Tak H, Chakraborty B, Carritt N, et al. The status of the Nebraska Healthcare Workforce: 2022 Update. Omaha, NE: UNMC Center for Health Policy; 2022.

29. Yang BK, Burcu M, Safer DJ, et al. Comparing nurse practitioner and physician prescribing of psychotropic medications for medicaid-insured youths. J Child Adolesc Psychopharmacol 2018;28(3):166–72.
30. Harrison JN, Cluxton-Keller F, Gross D. Antipsychotic medication prescribing trends in children and adolescents. J Pediatr Health Care 2012 Mar;26(2): 139–45. Available at: https://www.ncbi.nlm.nih.gov/pmc/articles/PMC3778027/.
31. Santosh PJ, Bell L, Fiori F, et al. Pediatric antipsychotic use and outcomes monitoring. J Child Adolesc Psychopharmacol 2017 Aug;27(6):546–54.
32. Reeves G, Anthony B. Multimodal treatments versus pharmacotherapy alone in children with psychiatric disorders: implications of access, effectiveness, and contextual treatment. Paediatr Drugs 2009;11(3):165–9.
33. Vitiello B. An update on publicly funded multisite trials in pediatric psychopharmacology. Child Adolesc Psychiatr Clin N Am 2006 Jan;15(1):1–12.
34. Zuckerbrot RA, Cheung A, Jensen PS, et al. Guidelines for Adolescent Depression in Primary Care (GLAD-PC): Part I. Practice preparation, identification, assessment, and initial management. Pediatrics 2018;141(3):e20174081.
35. Cheung AH, Zuckerbrot RA, Jensen PS, et al. Guidelines for Adolescent Depression in Primary Care (GLAD-PC): Part II. Treatment and ongoing management. Pediatrics 2018;141(3):e20174082.
36. Schrager SB. Integrating behavioral health into primary care. Fam Pract Manag 2021;28(3):3–4.
37. Horwitz SM, Storfer-Isser A, Kerker BD, et al. Barriers to the identification and management of psychosocial problems: changes from 2004 to 2013. Acad Pediatr 2015;15(6):613–20.
38. Raval GR, Doupnik SK. Closing the gap: improving access to mental health care through enhanced training in residency. Pediatrics 2017;139(1):e20163181.
39. Steele M, Zayed R, Davidson B, et al. Referral patterns and training needs in psychiatry among primary care physicians in canadian rural/remote areas. J Can Acad Child Adolesc Psychiatry 2012;21(2):111–23.
40. Zayed R, Davidson B, Nadeau L, et al. Canadian rural/remote primary care physicians perspectives on Child/Adolescent mental health care service delivery. J Can Acad Child Adolesc Psychiatry 2016;25(1):24–34.
41. McMillan JA, Land M, Leslie LK. Pediatric residency education and the behavioral and mental health crisis: a call to action. Pediatrics 2017;139(1):e20162141.
42. ACGME program requirements for graduate medical education in pediatrics. 2022. Available at: https://www.acgme.org/globalassets/pfassets/programrequirements/320_pediatrics_2023.pdf. Accessed February 14, 2024.
43. Child and Adolescent Psychiatry. American Board of Psychiatry and Neurology. 2024. Available at: https://abpn.org/become-certified/taking-a-subspecialty-exam/child-and-adolescent-psychiatry/#:~:text=Thetwoyearsoffull,theyearoftheexam. Accessed February 13, 2024.
44. Sawyer MG, Giesen F, Walter G. Child psychiatry curricula in undergraduate medical education. JAACAP 2008;47(2):139–47.
45. Schwartz RH, O'Laughlen MC, Kim J. Survey to child/adolescent psychiatry and developmental/behavioral pediatric training directors to expand psychiatric-mental health training to nurse practitioners. J Am Acad Nurse Pract 2017; 29(6):348–55.
46. Foy JM, Green CM, Earls MF, et al. Mental health competencies for pediatric practice. Pediatrics 2019;144(5):e20192757. https://doi.org/10.1542/peds.2019-2757.

47. Rubin R. It takes an average of 17 years for evidence to change practice—the burgeoning field of implementation science seeks to speed things up. JAMA 2023;329(16):1333–6.
48. Radhakrishnan L, Leeb RT, Bitsko RH, et al. Pediatric emergency department visits associated with mental health conditions before and during the COVID-19 Pandemic — United States, January 2019–January 2022. MMWR Morb Mortal Wkly Rep 2022;71:319–24.
49. Behavioral Health Workforce Education and training (BHWET) program for professionals. HRSA. Available at: https://www.hrsa.gov/grants/find-funding/HRSA-21-089. Accessed February 9, 2024.
50. Pediatric mental health care access. MCHB. 2024. Available at: https://mchb.hrsa.gov/programs-impact/programs/pediatric-mental-health-care-access. Accessed February 13, 2024.
51. FAQ: Primary care training and enhancement-residency training in mental and behavioral health (PCTE-RTMB). FAQ: Primary Care Training and Enhancement-Residency Training in Mental and Behavioral Health (PCTE-RTMB) | Bureau of Health Workforce. Available at: https://bhw.hrsa.gov/funding/apply-grant/faq-pcte-rtmb. Accessed February 10, 2024.
52. S.2938 - 117th congress (2021-2022): bipartisan safer communities act. Available at: https://www.congress.gov/bill/117th-congress/senate-bill/2938/text. Accessed June 25, 2022.
53. Oluyede L, Cochran AL, Wolfe M, et al. Addressing transportation barriers to health care during the COVID-19 pandemic: perspectives of care coordinators. Transp Res Part A Policy Pract 2022;159:157–68. Epub 2022 Mar 7. PMID: 35283561; PMCID: PMC8898700.
54. Telehealth policy changes after the COVID-19 public health emergency. telehealth.hhs.gov. 2023. Available at: https://telehealth.hhs.gov/providers/telehealth-policy/policy-changes-after-the-covid-19-public-health-emergency. Accessed February 14, 2024.
55. Bradley J, Jr J, Hastings S. Social justice advocacy in rural communities practical issues and implications. Counsel Psychol 2012;40:363–84.
56. Margolis K, Kelsay K, Talmi A, et al. A multidisciplinary, team-based teleconsultation approach to enhance child mental health services in rural pediatrics. J Educ Psychol Consult 2018;28(3):342–67.
57. Malas N, Klein E, Tengelitsch E, et al. Exploring the telepsychiatry experience: primary care provider perception of the Michigan Child Collaborative Care (MC3) program. Psychosomatics 2019;60(2):179–89.
58. Pediatric mental health care access program fact sheet. Available at: https://mchb.hrsa.gov/sites/default/files/mchb/about-us/pmhca-fact-sheet.pdf. Accessed January 26, 2024.
59. Lee CM, Yonek J, Lin B, et al. Systematic review: child psychiatry access program outcomes. JAACAP Open 2023;1(3):154–72. Epub 2023 Aug 1. PMID: 38189028; PMCID: PMC10769201.
60. Van Cleave J, Holifield C, Perrin JM. Primary care providers' use of a child psychiatry telephone support program. Acad Pediatr 2018;18(3):266–72. Epub 2017 Nov 29. PMID: 29197641.
61. Straus JH, Sarvet B. Behavioral health care for children: the Massachusetts child psychiatry access project. Health Aff 2014;33(12):2153–61.
62. Funded projects. MCHB. Available at: https://mchb.hrsa.gov/training/project_info.asp?id=777. Accessed January 27, 2024.

63. Primary care training and enhancement: physician assistant rural training in behavioral health (PCTE-PARB) program. HRSA. Available at: https://www.hrsa.gov/grants/find-funding/HRSA-24-019, Accessed February 8, 2024.
64. Primary care training and enhancement - residency training in mental and behavioral health (PCTE-RTMB). HRSA. Available at: https://www.hrsa.gov/grants/find-funding/HRSA-23-099. Accessed February 8, 2024.
65. Goodfellow A, Ulloa JG, Dowling PT, et al. Predictors of primary care physician practice location in underserved urban or rural areas in the United States: a systematic literature review. Acad Med 2016;91(9):1313–21.
66. Tools to help you. FREIDA. Available at: https://freida.ama-assn.org/. Accessed February 5, 2024.
67. Russell DJ, Wilkinson E, Petterson S, et al. Family medicine residencies: how rural training exposure in GME is associated with subsequent rural practice. J Grad Med Educ 2022;14(4):441–50.
68. Strong K, Gilbert M, Harris J, et al. Bipartisan Policy Center. Available at: https://bipartisanpolicy.org/. Accessed February 5, 2024.
69. Nielsen M, D'Agostino D, Gregory P. Addressing rural health challenges head on. Mo Med 2017;114(5):363–6. Available at: https://www.ncbi.nlm.nih.gov/pmc/articles/PMC6140198/pdf/ms114p0363.pdf.
70. Mann C, Striar A. How differences in medicaid, medicare, and commercial health insurance payment rates impact access, health equity, and cost. To the Point (Blog), Commonwealth Fund; 2022. https://doi.org/10.26099/c71g-322.
71. Drake RE, Latimer E. Lessons learned in developing community mental health care in North America. World J Psychiatry 2012;11(1):47–51. PMID: 22295009; PMCID: PMC3266763.
72. Community Mental Health Centers. CMS.gov. Available at: https://www.cms.gov/medicare/health-safety-standards/certification-compliance/community-mental-health-centers. Accessed February 10, 2024.
73. Wishon AA, Brown JD. Differences in services offered by certified community behavioral health clinics and community mental health centers. Psychiatr Serv 2023;74(4):411–4.
74. Certified Community Behavioral Health Clinics (CCBHCS). SAMHSA. 2023. Available at: https://www.samhsa.gov/certified-community-behavioral-health-clinics. Accessed February 10, 2024.
75. Certified community behavioral health clinics demonstration program: report to congress, 2018. ASPE. 2019. Available at: https://aspe.hhs.gov/reports/certified-community-behavioral-health-clinics-demonstration-program-report-congress-2018-0. Accessed February 10, 2024.
76. Quigley L. Incentive programs for physicians to practice in underserved areas: a nationwide snapshot. J Ambul Care Manage 2022;45(2):105–13. PMID: 35202027.
77. Whepley B. Western Kansas Hospital attracts doctors through focus on mission. University of Kansas School of Medicine-Wichita. 2014. Available at: https://www.kumc.edu/school-of-medicine/campuses/wichita/about/news/news-archive/lakin-feature-071114.html.
78. Quigley L. Whom do incentive program physicians serve? new measures for assessing program reach. J Ambul Care Manage 2022;45(4):266–78.

Opioid Use Disorder and Neonatal Opioid Withdrawal Syndrome in Rural Environments

Kristin Reese, MD*, Alison Holmes, MD, MPH

KEYWORDS

• Opioid use disorder • Pregnancy • Neonatal opioid withdrawal syndrome
• Neonatal abstinence syndrome • Rural

KEY POINTS

- Rural areas in the United States are disproportionally impacted by both opiod use disorder (OUD) during pregnancy and neonatal opioid withdrawal syndrome (NOWS).
- Pregnant persons with OUD in rural areas face many barriers to access care; innovative programs that integrate OUD treatment with obstetric care can improve outcomes.
- Increasing evidence supports the use of the Eat, Sleep, Console (ESC) assessment tool in management of NOWS; perinatal quality collaboratives have proven successful in implementing evidence-based care, such as ESC, in rural and community hospitals.
- Local, state, and federal agencies should prioritize policies and programs to meet the unique needs of rural communities.

INTRODUCTION

Over the last 2 decades, the United States has witnessed a dramatic increase in opioid use disorder (OUD) among pregnant persons, with a corresponding increase in neonatal opioid withdrawal syndrome (NOWS); both have disproportionately impacted rural areas.[1,2] People living in rural communities face numerous barriers to accessing care for OUD and NOWS. Access to prevention, treatment, and other support services is crucial for these birthing person-infant dyads, and solutions to improve care should be tailored to the unique needs of these rural communities.

DEFINITIONS

Opioid Use Disorder

OUD is diagnosed using criteria from the *Diagnostic and Statistical Manual of Mental Health Disorders*, Fifth Edition (DSM-5), and centers on "a problematic pattern of

Department of Pediatrics, Dartmouth Health Children's, 1 Medical Center Drive, Lebanon, NH 03766, USA
* Corresponding author.
E-mail address: Kristin.E.Reese@hitchcock.org

Pediatr Clin N Am 72 (2025) 37–52
https://doi.org/10.1016/j.pcl.2024.07.026 **pediatric.theclinics.com**
0031-3955/25/

opioid use leading to clinically significant impairment or distress." Substance use disorder (SUD) is similarly diagnosed, but more broadly includes alcohol, tobacco, and other nonprescribed substances.[3]

Neonatal Opioid Withdrawal Syndrome

Until recently, no standard definition of NOWS existed. In 2022, the US Department of Health and Human Services (HHS), along with experts in the field, led the development of a standard clinical definition for opioid withdrawal in infants, which includes prenatal exposure plus specific evidence-based clinical signs.[4,5] Traditionally, this syndrome has been called neonatal abstinence syndrome (NAS), a more general term that may include nonopioid exposure. In this article, the term NOWS is predominantly used in place of NAS.

EPIDEMIOLOGY

Hospital discharge data from the National Inpatient Sample (NIS) compiled by the Healthcare Cost and Utilization Project (HCUP) revealed that OUD documented at the delivery hospitalization quadrupled from 1999 to 2014,[2] and data from 2016 showed that rates of SUD-related deliveries among patients from rural areas was 59% higher than for patients living in urban areas.[6] As expected, the incidence of NOWS has similarly increased during the same time period,[7,8] disproportionally affecting rural areas.[9] Data from NIS/HCUP from 2004 to 2013 showed an increase in the national incidence of NOWS from 1.2 to 7.5 cases per 1000 hospital births among rural infants, versus from 1.4 to 4.8 cases among urban infants.[9] Updated data from 2010 to 2017 demonstrated an ongoing increase in the rates of both OUD at birth hospitalization and NOWS, with large state-level variation. NOWS rates ranged from 1.3 cases per 1000 birth hospitalizations in Nebraska to 53.5 cases per 1000 birth hospitalizations in West Virginia, with Maine, Vermont, Delaware, and Kentucky also exceeding 20 cases per 1000 birth hospitalizations. In rural areas, the rate of NOWS increased from 5.0 to 12.1 cases per 1000 birth hospitalizations, versus from 3.6 to 5.4 cases per 1000 birth hospitalizations in large metropolitan areas. In 2017, neonates with NOWS were significantly more likely to be non-Hispanic white, Medicaid-billed, and reside in zip codes with the lowest quartile of median income, and live in nonmetropolitan/rural counties (**Fig. 1**).[1]

OPIOID USE DISORDER IN PREGNANCY

Untreated OUD during pregnancy poses significant risk to both the pregnant person and the developing fetus, including overdose death, reluctance to obtain prenatal care, preterm birth, and low birth weight.[10] The American College of Obstetricians and Gynecologists (ACOG) recommends opioid agonist pharmacotherapy, also referred to as medication-assisted treatment (MAT), for pregnant persons with an OUD.[10] Methadone and buprenorphine, which target *mu*-opioid receptors, are both safe and effective options to treat OUD in pregnancy. Methadone can only be administered through designated opioid treatment programs, whereas buprenorphine can be prescribed in office-based settings.[11] Previously, buprenorphine could only be prescribed by providers who underwent specialized training and received a waiver from the Drug Enforcement Administration (DEA), but in 2023 the Consolidated Appropriations Act (also known as the Omnibus bill) removed the federal waiver requirement. Now all practitioners who have a current DEA registration that includes section III authority can prescribe buprenorphine for OUD if their practice is permitted by state law.[12] The decision to initiate methadone versus buprenorphine for OUD should be

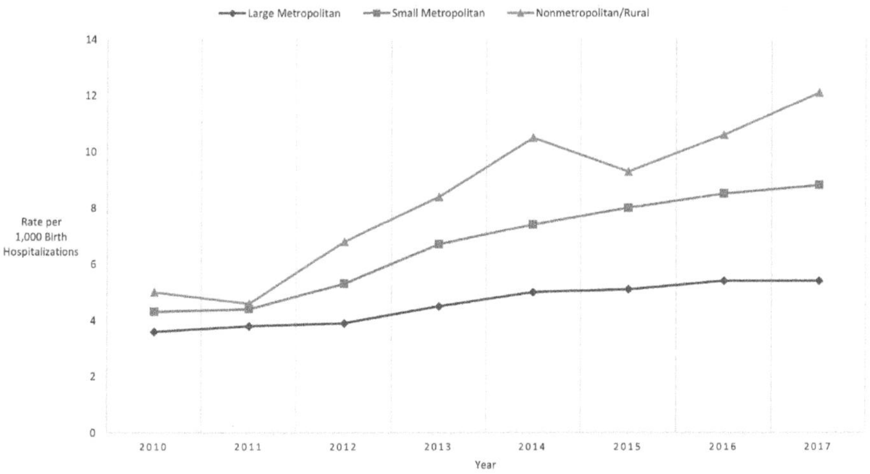

Fig. 1. Neonatal abstinence syndrome rates per 1,000 birth hospitalizations, urban versus rural residence, 2010-2017[a,b]. [a]Data from Hiral AH, Ko JY, Owens PL, et al. Neonatal abstinence syndrome and maternal opioid-related diagnoses in the US, 2010-2017. JAMA 2021;323(2):146-155. https://doi.org/10.1001/jama.2020.24991. Original source: Agency for Healthcare Research and Quality, Healthcare Cost and Utilization Project, national inpatient sample. [b]Based on a simplification of the US Department of Agricultures's urban influence codes to the following categories: large metropolitan counties (≥1 million residents in at least 1 urbanized area of a core-based statistical area), small metropolitan counties (50,000–999,999 residents in at least 1 urbanized area of a core-based statistical area), and nonmetropolitan/rural counties (micropolitan or noncore-based statistical area).

individualized based on multiple factors. There is emerging evidence that compared with methadone, the use of buprenorphine in pregnancy may be associated with lower risk of adverse neonatal outcomes, such as preterm birth, small for gestational age, and low birth weight (**Table 1**).[13]

Unfortunately, pregnant persons, especially those residing in rural areas, face many barriers in accessing OUD care.[14] In general, rural areas tend to have decreased access to opioid treatment programs and a decreased supply of buprenorphine-prescribing providers.[15–17] Acceptance of insurance, willingness to treat pregnant persons, and long wait times can pose additional barriers to care.[18,19] Pregnant persons in rural areas may also face challenges in accessing obstetric care itself. A recent report from the Center for Healthcare Quality and Payment Reform revealed that over the past decade, more than 200 rural hospitals in the United States have stopped delivering babies, and now 55% of rural hospitals in the United States do not even offer labor and delivery services.[20]

One way to improve access to OUD care involves assembling multidisciplinary care teams that integrate treatment for OUD with obstetric care.[21,22] Given high rates of comorbid mental health diagnoses, such as depression and post-traumatic stress disorder,[10] coordinating care with behavioral health providers further supports retention to treatment and improved outcomes.[23] A meta-analysis found that integrated obstetric and OUD care was effective in reducing substance use, although studies were small and heterogeneous.[24] A retrospective cohort study from a rural academic center in New England found that receiving integrated treatment was associated with increased engagement in obstetric care, lower risk for substance use at time of delivery, reduced

Table 1
Methadone vs buprenorphine for opioid use disorder

	Methadone	Both	Buprenorphine
Mechanism	• μ-opioid receptor full agonist		• μ-opioid receptor partial agonist
Administration	• Obtained at designated opioid treatment programs	• May be dispensed in hospital setting by physicians without waivers	• Can be prescribed in office-based setting by approved providers
Rural barriers	• Decreased access to opioid treatment programs	• Acceptance of insurance • Provider willing to treat pregnant persons • Long wait times	• Decreased supply of buprenorphine-prescribing providers
Risk of NOWS		• Yes	• May be associated with lower risk of adverse neonatal outcomes compared with methadone
Breastfeeding		• Safe • Present in low concentrations in human milk	

preterm birth rates, and shorter infant hospital stays. As the authors point out, "these findings have important implications for future prospective research and clinical program design especially in rural communities where access to obstetric and substance use care are impacted by lack of public transportation and economic vulnerability."[25]

SCREENING/TESTING

ACOG recommends universal screening for substance use at the first prenatal visit, using validated verbal screening tools, and a caring and nonjudgmental approach; if a pregnant person screens positive, follow-up should involve offering a brief intervention, and referring for specialized care as needed.[10] Urine drug testing is not routinely recommended, but it can be used to detect or confirm suspected substance use when performed with the patient's consent and in compliance with state law. Routine urine drug testing is controversial, as a positive result does not reveal information regarding timing, patterns, or severity of use, and there is a risk for false-negative and false-positive results.[10] Health care providers should also be aware of their laboratory's urine drug testing characteristics, as immunoassay techniques are the most common initial method used but can lead to false-positive results, especially for amphetamines and opioids.[26] Positive results from any immunoassay test should be considered presumptive, and confirmatory testing should be performed via gas-chromatography-mass spectrometry, or high-performance liquid chromatography.

Universal urine drug testing of birthing persons has been proposed as a means to increase detection of neonates at risk for NOWS, and to decrease bias in testing, but may be problematic for several reasons. One single-center cohort study at a community hospital that implemented universal maternal urine toxicology testing at delivery hospitalization found improved rates of detection of substance use compared with their risk-based testing protocol, with 20% of opioid-positive urine tests recorded in birthing people without screening risk factors.[27] These results are limited, however, because the study did not utilize a validated verbal screening tool in a comparison group. Universal testing approaches can also exacerbate racial and socioeconomic disparities in care. Studies have shown that Black women are reported to child protective services at a significantly higher rate than white women, despite similar rates of substance use among the 2 groups.[28,29]

The American Academy of Pediatrics (AAP) does not recommend routine newborn toxicology testing, unless it will inform clinical management.[30] Because of a lack of national guidelines to inform newborn toxicology testing, there is wide variability in practice, which risks inequities in care. At 1 academic center, the birthing persons of infants who underwent toxicology testing were significantly younger, identified as single, lived in the lowest income zip codes, and were less likely to identify as white.[31]

Similarly, the Academy of Breastfeeding Medicine (ABM) does not recommend routine urine drug testing to guide breast feeding decision making. If urine drug testing is pursued, results "must be interpreted within the clinical context including patient history and collateral information, and this should inform need for further confirmatory testing (eg, with gas chromatography)."[32]

PATHOPHYSIOLOGY OF NEONATAL OPIOID WITHDRAWAL SYNDROME

NOWS develops in the setting of chronic in utero exposure to opioids, and clinical presentation varies depending on the opioid type, as well as various factors associated with the birthing person, including other drug exposures, metabolism, and placental drug transfer.[30] Although higher cumulative in utero exposure to short-acting opioids may increase the risk of developing NOWS, the dose of maintenance opioids does not appear to alter the risk.[33] A meta-analysis of observational studies did not reveal a significant relationship between severity of NOWS and high- versus low-dose methadone.[34] Similarly, there is no dose-related relationship between buprenorphine and various neonatal outcomes, including NOWS severity.[35] Other factors that may increase the risk of NOWS include the birthing person's use of tobacco, selective serotonin reuptake inhibitors, and benzodiazepines.[33,36]

CLINICAL PRESENTATION OF NEONATAL OPIOID WITHDRAWAL SYNDROME

The clinical presentation of NOWS includes signs and symptoms of central nervous system irritability, autonomic over-reactivity, and gastrointestinal tract dysfunction; specific examples include tremor, feeding difficulty, diarrhea, and seizures.[37] The onset of symptoms varies depending on the half-life of the opioid, but generally occurs within the first 12 to 24 hours for a neonate exposed to a short-acting opioid like heroin, versus at 24 to 72 hours for long-acting methadone and buprenorphine (**Table 2**).[37,38]

NEONATAL OPIOID WITHDRAWAL SYNDROME MANAGEMENT

The management of NOWS involves a period of observation, combined with nonpharmacologic care (such as parental engagement, rooming-in, skin-to-skin, low-stimulation environment, and breastfeeding), and in severe cases the addition of medication to improve signs of withdrawal.[30] There is a lack of strong evidence to support a standard approach to management of NOWS, resulting in wide variability of inpatient care, length of stay (LOS), and cost.[39–41] A 2015 survey of hospitals in the Better Outcomes Through Research For Newborns (BORN) network found significant variation in observation periods for short- and long-acting opioids, pharmacologic and

Table 2
Clinical presentation of neonatal opioid withdrawal syndrome

Central Nervous System Irritability	Autonomic Over-reactivity	Gastrointestinal Tract Dysfunction
• Tremors • Increased wakefulness/ decreased sleep • Increased muscle tone • Hyperactive reflexes • Exaggerated Moro reflex • Seizures	• Increased sweating • Nasal stuffiness • Fever • Frequent yawning and sneezing	• Feeding difficulties • Uncoordinated suck • Vomiting • Diarrhea/loose stools

nonpharmacologic management, and breastfeeding practices.[40] Data from the Pediatric Health Information System also reveal wide variation in hospital rates of pharmacotherapy for management of NOWS (ranging from 13%-90%) and the type of medication chosen for management of withdrawal.[39,41]

Nonpharmacologic Management

All infants with chronic in utero exposure to opioids should be observed in the hospital for at least 72 hours to monitor for signs and symptoms of withdrawal. There is limited evidence to guide observation periods, but generally the recommendation is 3 days for infants exposed to short-acting opioids, versus 4 to 7 days for long-acting opioids like buprenorphine and methadone.[30]

Historically, the Finnegan Neonatal Abstinence Scoring Tool, or a modified version of it, has been used to assess the severity of neonatal withdrawal symptoms and guide decisions on pharmacologic treatment.[42] Because of concern that this assessment tool leads to highly variable and potentially unnecessary opioid treatment for babies with NOWS, in 2014 Grossman and colleagues proposed a novel approach called Eat, Sleep, Console (ESC). This care focuses on nonpharmacologic interventions, including parental presence, swaddling/holding, feeding on demand, and a low-stimulation environment to promote essential newborn functions-namely, the baby's ability to eat sufficient quantities, to sleep uninterrupted for at least 1 hour, and to be consoled within 10 minutes.[43,44]

A recent cluster-randomized controlled trial at 26 US hospitals that compared the ESC approach to usual care found a significant decrease in time until infants were medically ready for discharge by a mean of 6.7 days among the ESC group (8.2 versus 14.9 days; adjusted mean difference, 6.7 days; 95% confidence interval [CI], 4.7–8.8); infants in the ESC group were also treated with opioids less often (19.5% among ESC group versus 52% in usual care group), without increasing any adverse safety outcomes through 3 months of age.[45] This study included academic medical centers and community hospitals, and selected sites that were geographically diverse. Given that the ESC approach emphasizes parental involvement in care, and is often less resource intensive, it is primed for success in rural communities.

Pharmacologic Management

If an infant continues to display severe withdrawal symptoms despite optimization of nonpharmacologic interventions, pharmacologic therapy should be considered. There is variability surrounding decisions to initiate pharmacotherapy. For institutions using the Finnegan or similar scoring tool, pharmacologic treatment is generally initiated when single or serial withdrawal scores exceed a prespecified threshold.[37] For infants being monitored with the ESC Care Tool, the approach often involves a multidisciplinary team huddle to discuss pharmacologic treatment if the infant has issues eating, sleeping, or consoling despite maximizing nonpharmacologic interventions.[46] The first-line agent for management of neonatal opioid withdrawal symptoms is an opioid.[37,47] Most commonly oral morphine is used, but methadone and buprenorphine are also utilized, and there is insufficient evidence to recommend 1 agent over another.[48] However, across multiple studies, buprenorphine was consistently associated with shorter LOS.[47–49]

Perinatal Quality Collaboratives

Rural regions in the United States are often served by community hospitals, and many infants with NOWS are transferred from community hospitals to academic medical centers, which can disrupt maternal-infant bonding and family support. In 1 observational study of 2 rural community hospitals that used a standardized care protocol for assessment and treatment of NOWS, there was no significant difference between mean LOS, LOS due to NOWS, and duration of NOWS treatment in the community setting compared with academic practice settings.[50]

A strategy to improve care among rural and community hospitals involves utilizing Perinatal Quality Collaboratives (PQCs), which are "state or multistate networks of teams working to improve the quality of care for mothers and babies."[51] PQCs are primed to leverage their strengths to support the creation and dissemination of rural birthing person and infant health improvements.[52] The Northern New England Perinatal Quality Improvement Network (NNEPQIN) is 1 such collaborative that includes most of the birth hospitals in New Hampshire, Vermont, and Maine.[53] In 2018, NNEPQIN utilized their regional network to implement the ESC care tool in hospitals across the region, many of which are located in rural areas.[54]

From 2017 to 2019, the Massachusetts state Perinatal-Neonatal Quality Improvement Network (PNQIN) successfully implemented an ESC NOWS Care Tool across multiple hospitals, resulting in a decrease in pharmacotherapy and LOS, without an increase in short-term adverse events; sustained changes were noted in both tertiary and community hospital settings.[46] Similarly, from 2017 to 2019, the Colorado Hospitals Substance Exposed Newborn Quality Improvement Collaborative (CHoSEN QIC) standardized the care of opioid exposed newborns (OENs) among birthing hospitals in the state, which included using the ESC approach, and also found a decrease in pharmacotherapy and LOS.[55] A secondary analysis of this quality improvement initiative investigated disparities in care by Hispanic ethnicity, and found that Hispanic newborns experienced a delay of 3 calendar quarters in achieving decreased LOS, and a 1-quarter delay to lower pharmacotherapy compared with non-Hispanic newborns.[56] This highlights the ability of quality improvement networks to evaluate health care disparities and mitigate them by developing initiatives that are tailored to the unique needs of diverse populations, including rural populations (**Fig. 2**).

Telehealth

Telehealth services provide another opportunity for improving health in rural areas. HCUP data from 2004 to 2013 revealed that compared with their urban peers, rural infants and birthing persons with opioid-related diagnoses were more likely to be transferred to another hospital following delivery.[9] Hospital transfer may increase stress during what can already be a challenging time for new parents. Telemedicine has emerged as a feasible option to improve quality of care for rural communities, including perinatal and newborn care.[57] Televideo educational models have also been utilized to train rural primary care providers in OUD management, which could easily be translated to NOWS care.[58]

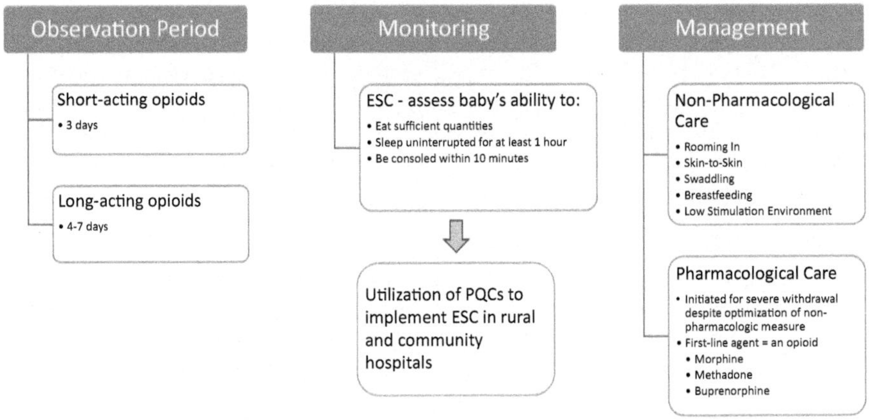

Fig. 2. Management of NOWS.

BREASTFEEDING

The Academy of Breastfeeding Medicine (ABM), AAP, and ACOG all support breastfeeding among people with OUD who are stable in recovery and receiving treatment, are not using nonprescribed substances, and have no other contraindications to breastfeeding.[10,32,59] Breastfeeding is safe and should be encouraged for caregivers who take methadone or buprenorphine, as both substances are present in relatively low concentrations in human milk, and breastfeeding may help reduce the severity of NOWS.[30,32] In addition, new ABM guidelines released in 2023 support breastfeeding initiation among persons who discontinue nonprescribed substance use by or during the delivery hospitalization, whereas previous recommendations discouraged breastfeeding with any nonprescribed substance use in the 30 to 90 days before delivery.[32] This updated recommendation was informed in part by a retrospective cohort study that found nonprescribed substance use at delivery had the strongest association with ongoing nonprescribed use postpartum, compared with earlier time points in pregnancy.[60]

Despite known benefits of breastfeeding for babies with NOWS, the rate of breastfeeding initiation and continuation among persons with OUD remains lower than the general population, reasons for which are not fully understood.[30,61] Reported barriers from postpartum persons with OUD include concern about infant exposure to medications or substances, lack of support and education, and long neonatal intensive care unit (NICU) stays.[62,63] At 1 urban center, hospital-level factors were the greatest predictor of breastfeeding initiation among persons with OUD; the authors speculated that expanded breastfeeding eligibility criteria, quality improvement efforts to improve outcomes for babies with NOWS, and increased breastfeeding education led to increased breastfeeding rates at their institution over a decade.[64]

Literature specifically examining breastfeeding with OUD in rural areas is lacking. In general, infants in rural areas are less likely to ever breastfeed compared with infants living in urban areas.[65] Birthing persons with lower socioeconomic status, who are younger, and those with high school education or less are less likely to breastfeed,[65] and many of these factors are more prevalent in rural areas compared with urban ones. Numerous barriers to breastfeeding in rural environments also exist, including lack of breastfeeding assistance, time constraints and early return to work, and lack of continued support.[66,67] Public health efforts to support breastfeeding in rural areas should be a priority, especially among opioid-exposed newborns.

DISCHARGE AND FOLLOW-UP

Discharge planning to prepare for a safe transition to home is an important piece of care for the birthing person-infant dyad, and ideally should be managed by a multidisciplinary team of pediatric and obstetric providers, nursing, lactation, social work, and care management.

Birthing persons with OUD should continue opioid agonist therapy postpartum, especially in light of an increased risk for relapse during this time period compared with during pregnancy.[68] Changes in methadone or buprenorphine dosage are not routinely needed, but dosage reductions should be titrated to signs and symptoms of sedation.[10] The immediate postpartum period can be a time of increased stress because of the demands of caring for a new baby, sleep deprivation, concerns about child custody, and the possibility of loss of insurance and access to treatment. Medicaid insurance covers about 4 in 10 births in the United States, and most US states have implemented or are planning to implement extended Medicaid coverage to 12 months postpartum; however, in Arkansas and Wisconsin pregnancy-related Medicaid coverage only lasts 60 and 90 days postpartum, respectively.[69] Screening for postpartum depression and other comorbid mental health conditions should also be a routine part of follow-up care, with access to psychosocial support services if indicated.[10]

Infants with NOWS should have their first primary care follow-up appointment within 24 to 48 hours of hospital discharge, to monitor for any new or continued signs of withdrawal, and to assess feeding and weight gain. There is no specific timeline for additional follow-up visits, but they should be adjusted to meet the unique needs of the birthing person-infant dyad.[30]

Plan of Safe Care

Per the federal Child Abuse Prevention and Treatment Act (CAPTA), all opioid-exposed newborns require a Plan of Safe Care (POSC), sometimes also called a Plan of Supportive Care. The goal of the POSC is to increase access to care and treatment for infants and families affected by substance use, which can be tailored to specific family needs. Because CAPTA does not mandate which state agency is responsible for planning and implementation of the POSC, there is variation from state to state. Pediatric providers should be aware of their local policies and expectations.[30,70]

Early Intervention

The dyad should be offered additional services, including early intervention programs. Opioid-exposed infants are at increased risk for developmental and behavioral concerns, although the neurodevelopmental effects of prenatal opioid exposure itself have proved impossible to separate from confounding socioeconomic, genetic, and environmental variables.[30,71] Unfortunately, many eligible newborns never receive early intervention services. One single-center retrospective cohort study found that fewer than half of eligible infants with NOWS were enrolled in early intervention services after hospital discharge. This study also found that the odds of early intervention referral were about twice as high among infants discharged to a biological parent compared with foster care, and longer hospital stays had the strongest association with early intervention enrollment.[72]

Challenges in accessing early intervention services may be exacerbated by living in a rural area, secondary to issues with the referral process and services available. A Kentucky study found that families living in high-poverty areas that were also rural accessed fewer services compared with their urban counterparts.[73] From a nationally representative sample of families receiving early intervention services, families from rural areas were more likely to receive a wait-and-see response from their health care provider to symptoms, subsequently delaying access to early identification and services.[74] From a qualitative study examining the early intervention referral process in rural Montana, families reported feeling that rurality related to their experience of high turnover rate, lack of access to services or professional knowledge about specific conditions, and long travel distance to access services.[75]

Home Nurse Visitation Programs

Referral to home nurse visitation programs can be another helpful resource for families. The Maternal, Infant, and Early Childhood Home Visiting (MIECHV) Program, for example, supports home visiting programs for new and expectant parents who live in communities that are at higher risk for poor health outcomes. In fiscal year 2022, the MIECHIV Program served all 50 states, and 60% of all counties served were rural.[76] However, structural barriers exist to engage and serve rural communities, including struggles to recruit and retain highly qualified staff, long travel times, lack of childcare, and lack of community trust (**Fig. 3**).[77]

PUBLIC POLICY

There is wide variability among states regarding reporting of NAS/NOWS. A 2013 to 2017 study found that 6 states (Arizona, Florida, Georgia, Kentucky, Tennessee, and Virginia) mandated reporting of NOWS cases from medical facilities to state health departments. These 6 states varied in their definition of NOWS, highlighting the need for a standardized case definition. How the surveillance data were used also varied; during interviews, however, state officials consistently noted that "mandated reporting of NAS was enacted to (1) gain a more precise understanding of the incidence of NAS in their state, (2) better characterize the impact of the opioid crisis in their state, (3) identify specific communities or geographic areas more severely affected by opioids and NAS, and (4) inform programs and services."[78]

A study using the state-wide surveillance system in Tennessee found high rates of NOWS, especially in the eastern, more mountainous counties in the state.[79] Similarly, a study performed in West Virginia utilized a real-time statewide surveillance system to demonstrate the state's rate of NOWS and its geographic distribution. Nearly half of people in West Virginia live in rural areas, and the authors found the rate of NOWS

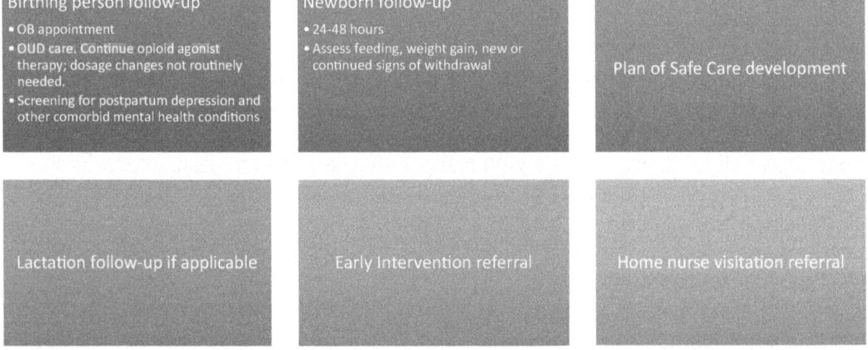

Fig. 3. Discharge to do list.

in the state to be nearly tenfold the national estimate.[80] These and other population-based surveillance systems often highlight the vulnerability of rural communities, and can be used to inform evidence-based interventions to improve outcomes for OUD and NOWS in high-risk areas.[81] Utilization of real-time data has the additional advantage of potential for guiding targeted intervention in a more timely manner.

SUMMARY

Over the last 2 decades, rural communities in the United States have experienced a steep rise in OUD during pregnancy, with a parallel increase in NOWS. These communities often encounter multiple barriers in accessing care, and the development of innovative programs helps address these gaps. The delivery of high-quality, evidence-based prevention, treatment, and support services is crucial for this vulnerable population. To improve the health of rural birthing person-infant dyads affected by OUD and NOWS, continued advocacy, research, and policy efforts must focus on the unique needs of rural communities in the United States.

CLINICS CARE POINTS

- Rural areas in the United States are disproportionally impacted by OUD during pregnancy and NOWS, and patients face barriers to accessing care.
- Per ACOG recommendation, universal screening for substance use should occur at the first prenatal visit, using a caring and nonjudgmental approach. Pregnant persons with OUD should receive opioid agonist pharmacotherapy, although access to this care in rural areas can be challenging.
- Increasing evidence supports the use of ESC in management of NOWS; perinatal quality collaboratives have proven successful in implementing evidence-based care, such as ESC, in rural and community hospitals.
- Breastfeeding should be encouraged among people with OUD who are stable in recovery and receiving treatment, are not using nonprescribed substances, and have no other contraindications to breastfeeding.
- Local, state, and federal agencies should prioritize policies and programs to meet the unique needs of rural communities.

DISCLOSURE

The authors have nothing to disclose.

REFERENCES

1. Hirai AH, Ko JY, Owens PL, et al. Neonatal abstinence syndrome and maternal opioid-related diagnoses in the US, 2010-2017. JAMA 2021;325(2):146–55. https://doi.org/10.1001/jama.2020.24991.
2. Haight SC, Ko JY, Tong VT, et al. Opioid use disorder documented at delivery hospitalization — United States, 1999–2014. MMWR Morb Mortal Wkly Rep 2018;67(31):845–9. https://doi.org/10.15585/mmwr.mm6731a1.
3. American Psychiatric Association. Diagnostic and statistical manual of mental disorders: DSM-5TM. 5th Edition. Washington, DC: American Psychiatric Publishing, Inc; 2013. https://doi.org/10.1176/appi.books.9780890425596.

4. Health (OASH) O of the AS for. HHS announces a standard clinical definition for opioid withdrawal in infants. 2022. Available at: https://www.hhs.gov/about/news/2022/01/31/hhs-announces-standard-clinical-definition-for-opioid-withdrawal-in-infants.html. Accessed February 28, 2024.
5. Jilani SM, Jones HE, Grossman M, et al. Standardizing the clinical definition of opioid withdrawal in the neonate. J Pediatr 2022;243:33–9.e1. https://doi.org/10.1016/j.jpeds.2021.12.021.
6. Obstetric delivery inpatient stays involving substance use disorders and related clinical outcomes, 2016 #254. Available at: https://hcup-us.ahrq.gov/reports/statbriefs/sb254-Delivery-Hospitalizations-Substance-Use-Clinical-Outcomes-2016.jsp. Accessed December 13, 2023.
7. Ko JY. Incidence of neonatal abstinence syndrome — 28 states, 1999–2013. MMWR Morb Mortal Wkly Rep 2016;65. https://doi.org/10.15585/mmwr.mm6531a2.
8. Patrick SW, Davis MM, Lehmann CU, et al. Increasing incidence and geographic distribution of neonatal abstinence syndrome: United States 2009 to 2012. J Perinatol 2015;35(8):650–5. https://doi.org/10.1038/jp.2015.36.
9. Villapiano NLG, Winkelman TNA, Kozhimannil KB, et al. Rural and urban differences in neonatal abstinence syndrome and maternal opioid use, 2004 to 2013. JAMA Pediatr 2017;171(2):194–6. https://doi.org/10.1001/jamapediatrics.2016.3750.
10. Committee opinion no. 711: opioid use and opioid use disorder in pregnancy. Obstet Gynecol 2017;130(2):e81. https://doi.org/10.1097/AOG.0000000000002235.
11. National Academies of Sciences. Division H and M, Policy B on HS, Disorder C on MAT for OU, Mancher M, Leshner AI. Summary. In: Medications for opioid use disorder save lives. National Academies Press (US); 2019. Available at: https://www.ncbi.nlm.nih.gov/books/NBK541390/. Accessed December 19, 2023.
12. Waiver Elimination (MAT Act). 2023. Available at: https://www.samhsa.gov/medications-substance-use-disorders/waiver-elimination-mat-act. Accessed January 21, 2024.
13. Suarez EA, Huybrechts KF, Straub L, et al. Buprenorphine versus methadone for opioid use disorder in pregnancy. N Engl J Med 2022;387(22):2033–44. https://doi.org/10.1056/NEJMoa2203318.
14. Henkhaus LE, Buntin MB, Henderson SC, et al. Disparities in receipt of medications for opioid use disorder among pregnant women. Subst Abuse 2022;43(1):508–13. https://doi.org/10.1080/08897077.2021.1949664.
15. Mitchell P, Samsel S, Curtin KM, et al. Geographic disparities in access to medication for opioid use disorder across US census tracts based on treatment utilization behavior. Soc Sci Med 2022;302:114992. https://doi.org/10.1016/j.socscimed.2022.114992.
16. Rosenblatt RA, Andrilla CHA, Catlin M, et al. Geographic and specialty distribution of US physicians trained to treat opioid use disorder. Ann Fam Med 2015;13(1):23–6. https://doi.org/10.1370/afm.1735.
17. Joudrey PJ, Kolak M, Lin Q, et al. Assessment of community-level vulnerability and access to medications for opioid use disorder. JAMA Netw Open 2022;5(4):e227028. https://doi.org/10.1001/jamanetworkopen.2022.7028.
18. Patrick SW, Buntin MB, Martin PR, et al. Barriers to accessing treatment for pregnant women with opioid use disorder in Appalachian states. Subst Abuse 2019;40(3):356–62. https://doi.org/10.1080/08897077.2018.1488336.
19. Patrick SW, Richards MR, Dupont WD, et al. Association of pregnancy and insurance status with treatment access for opioid use disorder. JAMA Netw Open 2020;3(8):e2013456. https://doi.org/10.1001/jamanetworkopen.2020.13456.

20. Center for Healthcare Quality & Payment Reform. Addressing the crisis in rural maternity care. Available at: https://ruralhospitals.chqpr.org/downloads/Rural_Maternity_Care_Crisis.pdf. Accessed March 1, 2024.
21. Goler NC, Armstrong MA, Taillac CJ, et al. Substance abuse treatment linked with prenatal visits improves perinatal outcomes: a new standard. J Perinatol 2008; 28(9):597–603. https://doi.org/10.1038/jp.2008.70.
22. Saia KA, Schiff D, Wachman EM, et al. Caring for pregnant women with opioid use disorder in the USA: expanding and improving treatment. Curr Obstet Gynecol Rep 2016;5(3):257–63. https://doi.org/10.1007/s13669-016-0168-9.
23. Goodman DJ, Milliken CU, Theiler RN, et al. A multidisciplinary approach to the treatment of co-occurring opioid use disorder and posttraumatic stress disorder in pregnancy: a case report. J Dual Diagn 2015;11(0):248–57. https://doi.org/10.1080/15504263.2015.1104484.
24. Milligan K, Niccols A, Sword W, et al. Birth outcomes for infants born to women participating in integrated substance abuse treatment programs: a meta-analytic review. In: Database of abstracts of reviews of effects (DARE): quality-assessed reviews [internet]. (UK): Centre for Reviews and Dissemination; 2011. Available at: https://www.ncbi.nlm.nih.gov/books/NBK91756/. Accessed February 27, 2024.
25. Goodman DJ, Saunders EC, Frew JR, et al. Integrated vs nonintegrated treatment for perinatal opioid use disorder: retrospective cohort study. Am J Obstet Gynecol MFM 2022;4(1):100489. https://doi.org/10.1016/j.ajogmf.2021.100489.
26. Moeller KE, Lee KC, Kissack JC. Urine drug screening: practical guide for clinicians. Mayo Clin Proc 2008;83(1):66–76. https://doi.org/10.4065/83.1.66.
27. Wexelblatt SL, Ward LP, Torok K, et al. Universal maternal drug testing in a high-prevalence region of prescription opiate abuse. J Pediatr 2015;166(3):582–6. https://doi.org/10.1016/j.jpeds.2014.10.004.
28. Roberts SCM, Nuru-Jeter A. Universal screening for alcohol and drug use and racial disparities in Child Protective Services reporting. J Behav Health Serv Res 2012;39(1):3–16. https://doi.org/10.1007/s11414-011-9247-x.
29. Chasnoff IJ, Landress HJ, Barrett ME. The prevalence of illicit-drug or alcohol use during pregnancy and discrepancies in mandatory reporting in Pinellas County, Florida. N Engl J Med 1990;322(17):1202–6. https://doi.org/10.1056/NEJM199004263221706.
30. Patrick SW, Barfield WD, Poindexter BB, et al. Neonatal opioid withdrawal syndrome. Pediatrics 2020;146(5). https://doi.org/10.1542/peds.2020-029074. e2020029074.
31. Perlman NC, Cantonwine DE, Smith NA. Toxicology testing in a newborn ICU: does social profiling play a role? Hosp Pediatr 2021;11(9):e179–83. https://doi.org/10.1542/hpeds.2020-005765.
32. Harris M, Schiff DM, Saia K, et al. Academy of breastfeeding medicine clinical protocol #21: breastfeeding in the setting of substance use and substance use disorder (revised 2023). Breastfeed Med 2023;18(10):715–33. https://doi.org/10.1089/bfm.2023.29256.abm.
33. Patrick SW, Dudley J, Martin PR, et al. Prescription opioid epidemic and infant outcomes. Pediatrics 2015;135(5):842–50. https://doi.org/10.1542/peds.2014-3299.
34. Cleary BJ, Donnelly J, Strawbridge J, et al. Methadone dose and neonatal abstinence syndrome—systematic review and meta-analysis. Addiction 2010;105(12): 2071–84. https://doi.org/10.1111/j.1360-0443.2010.03120.x.
35. Jones HE, Dengler E, Garrison A, et al. Neonatal outcomes and their relationship to maternal buprenorphine dose during pregnancy. Drug Alcohol Depend 2014; 134:414–7. https://doi.org/10.1016/j.drugalcdep.2013.11.006.

36. Sanlorenzo LA, Cooper WO, Dudley JA, et al. Increased severity of neonatal abstinence syndrome associated with concomitant antenatal opioid and benzodiazepine exposure. Hosp Pediatr 2019;9(8):569–75. https://doi.org/10.1542/hpeds.2018-0227.
37. Hudak ML, Tan RC, et al, The Committee on Drugs. Neonatal drug withdrawal. Pediatrics 2012;129(2):e540–60. https://doi.org/10.1542/peds.2011-3212.
38. Zelson C, Rubio E, Wasserman E. Neonatal narcotic addiction: 10 year observation. Pediatrics 1971;48(2):178–89. https://doi.org/10.1542/peds.48.2.178.
39. Milliren CE, Gupta M, Graham DA, et al. Hospital variation in neonatal abstinence syndrome incidence, treatment modalities, resource use, and costs across pediatric hospitals in the United States, 2013 to 2016. Hosp Pediatr 2018;8(1):15–20. https://doi.org/10.1542/hpeds.2017-0077.
40. Bogen DL, Whalen B, Kair LR, et al. Wide variation found in care of opioid-exposed newborns. Acad Pediatr 2017;17(4):374–80. https://doi.org/10.1016/j.acap.2016.10.003.
41. Patrick SW, Kaplan HC, Passarella M, et al. Variation in treatment of neonatal abstinence syndrome in US children's hospitals, 2004–2011. J Perinatol 2014;34(11):867–72. https://doi.org/10.1038/jp.2014.114.
42. Finnegan LP, Connaughton JF, Kron RE, et al. Neonatal abstinence syndrome: assessment and management. Addict Dis 1975;2(1–2):141–58.
43. Grossman MR, Berkwitt AK, Osborn RR, et al. An initiative to improve the quality of care of infants with neonatal abstinence syndrome. Pediatrics 2017;139(6):e20163360. https://doi.org/10.1542/peds.2016-3360.
44. Grossman MR, Lipshaw MJ, Osborn RR, et al. A novel approach to assessing infants with neonatal abstinence syndrome. Hosp Pediatr 2018;8(1):1–6. https://doi.org/10.1542/hpeds.2017-0128.
45. Young LW, Ounpraseuth ST, Merhar SL, et al. Eat, Sleep, Console approach or usual care for neonatal opioid withdrawal. N Engl J Med 2023;388(25):2326–37. https://doi.org/10.1056/NEJMoa2214470.
46. Wachman EM, Houghton M, Melvin P, et al. A quality improvement initiative to implement the eat, sleep, console neonatal opioid withdrawal syndrome care tool in Massachusetts' PNQIN collaborative. J Perinatol 2020;40(10):1560–9. https://doi.org/10.1038/s41372-020-0733-y.
47. Zankl A, Martin J, Davey JG, et al. Opioid treatment for opioid withdrawal in newborn infants. Cochrane Database Syst Rev 2021;2021(7):CD002059. https://doi.org/10.1002/14651858.CD002059.pub4.
48. Wachman EM, Schiff DM, Silverstein M. Neonatal abstinence syndrome: advances in diagnosis and treatment. JAMA 2018;319(13):1362–74. https://doi.org/10.1001/jama.2018.2640.
49. Disher T, Gullickson C, Singh B, et al. Pharmacological treatments for neonatal abstinence syndrome. JAMA Pediatr 2019;173(3):234–43. https://doi.org/10.1001/jamapediatrics.2018.5044.
50. Friedman H, Parkinson G, Tighiouart H, et al. Pharmacologic treatment of infants with neonatal abstinence syndrome in community hospitals compared to academic medical centers. J Perinatol 2018;38(12):1651–6. https://doi.org/10.1038/s41372-018-0230-8.
51. Perinatal Quality Collaboratives. CDC. 2023. Available at: https://www.cdc.gov/reproductivehealth/maternalinfanthealth/pqc.htm. Accessed January 22, 2024.
52. Main EK, Sakowski C. How state perinatal quality collaboratives can improve rural maternity care. Clin Obstet Gynecol 2022;65(4):848–55. https://doi.org/10.1097/GRF.0000000000000748.

53. Northern New England Perinatal Quality Improvement Network. 2017. Available at: https://www.nnepqin.org/. Accessed January 22, 2024.
54. Whalen B., MacMillan K., Flanagan V., et al., NNEPQIN NAS initiative: implementation of eat, sleep, console care tool across a regional neonatal quality improvement network. In: Proceedings from the 2019 annual meeting of the pediatric academic societies. April 24-May 1, 2019. Baltimore, MD.
55. Hwang SS, Weikel B, Adams J, et al. The Colorado Hospitals Substance Exposed Newborn Quality Improvement Collaborative. Standardization of care for opioid-exposed newborns shortens length of stay and reduces number of infants requiring opiate therapy. Hosp Pediatr 2020;10(9):783–91. https://doi.org/10.1542/hpeds.2020-0032.
56. Weikel BW, Palau MA, Hwang SS. Ethnic disparities in the care of opioid-exposed newborns in Colorado birthing hospitals. Hosp Pediatr 2021;11(11):1190–8. https://doi.org/10.1542/hpeds.2021-005824.
57. Marcin JP, Shaikh U, Steinhorn RH. Addressing health disparities in rural communities using telehealth. Pediatr Res 2016;79(1):169–76. https://doi.org/10.1038/pr.2015.192.
58. Komaromy M, Duhigg D, Metcalf A, et al. Project ECHO (Extension for Community Healthcare Outcomes): a new model for educating primary care providers about treatment of substance use disorders. Subst Abuse 2016;37(1):20–4. https://doi.org/10.1080/08897077.2015.1129388.
59. Meek JY, Noble L. Section on breastfeeding. policy statement: breastfeeding and the use of human milk. Pediatrics 2022;150(1). https://doi.org/10.1542/peds.2022-057988. e2022057988.
60. Harris M, Joseph K, Hoeppner B, et al. A retrospective cohort study examining the utility of perinatal urine toxicology testing to guide breastfeeding initiation. J Addict Med 2021;15(4):311–7. https://doi.org/10.1097/ADM.0000000000000761.
61. Clark RRS. Breastfeeding in women on opioid maintenance therapy: a review of policy and practice. J Midwifery Wom Health 2019;64(5):545–58. https://doi.org/10.1111/jmwh.12982.
62. Yonke N, Jimenez EY, Leeman L, et al. Breastfeeding motivators and barriers in women receiving medications for opioid use disorder. Breastfeed Med 2020;15(1):17–23. https://doi.org/10.1089/bfm.2019.0122.
63. Hicks J, Morse E, Wyant DK. Barriers and facilitators of breastfeeding reported by postpartum women in methadone maintenance therapy. Breastfeed Med 2018;13(4):259–65. https://doi.org/10.1089/bfm.2017.0130.
64. Schiff DM, Wachman EM, Philipp B, et al. Examination of hospital, maternal, and infant characteristics associated with breastfeeding initiation and continuation among opioid-exposed mother-infant dyads. Breastfeed Med 2018;13(4):266–74. https://doi.org/10.1089/bfm.2017.0172.
65. CDC. Breastfeeding rates: national immunization survey (NIS). Centers for Disease Control and Prevention; 2023. Available at: https://www.cdc.gov/breastfeeding/data/nis_data/index.htm. Accessed January 4, 2024.
66. Flower KB, Willoughby M, Cadigan RJ, et al. understanding breastfeeding initiation and continuation in rural communities: a combined qualitative/quantitative approach. Matern Child Health J 2008;12(3):402–14. https://doi.org/10.1007/s10995-007-0248-6.
67. Goodman LR, Majee W, Olsberg JE, et al. Breastfeeding barriers and support in a rural setting. MCN Am J Matern Nurs 2016;41(2):98. https://doi.org/10.1097/NMC.0000000000000212.

68. Gopman S. Prenatal and postpartum care of women with substance use disorders. Obstet Gynecol Clin 2014;41(2):213–28. https://doi.org/10.1016/j.ogc.2014.02.004.
69. Published: Medicaid postpartum coverage extension tracker. KFF; 2024. Available at: https://www.kff.org/medicaid/issue-brief/medicaid-postpartum-coverage-extension-tracker/. Accessed January 29, 2024.
70. NOWS – planning for maternal and infant discharge. Available at: https://www.aap.org/en/patient-care/opioids/maternal-infant-health-and-opioid-use-program/recovery-friendly-pediatric-care/nows–planning-for-maternal-and-infant-discharge/. Accessed February 14, 2024.
71. Benninger KL, McAllister JM, Merhar SL. Neonatal opioid withdrawal syndrome: an update on developmental outcomes. Clin Perinatol 2023;50(1):17–29. https://doi.org/10.1016/j.clp.2022.10.007.
72. Peacock-Chambers E, Leyenaar JK, Foss S, et al. Early intervention referral and enrollment among infants with neonatal abstinence syndrome. J Dev Behav Pediatr JDBP 2019;40(6):441–50. https://doi.org/10.1097/DBP.0000000000000679.
73. Level and intensity of early intervention services for infants and toddlers with disabilities: the impact of child, family, system, and community-level factors on service provision. 2009. Available at: https://journals.sagepub.com/doi/10.1177/1053815109331914. Accessed February 13, 2024.
74. Barnard-Brak L, Morales-Alemán MM, Tomeny K, et al. Rural and racial/ethnic differences in children receiving early intervention services. Fam Community Health 2021;44(1):52. https://doi.org/10.1097/FCH.0000000000000285.
75. Decker KB, Williams ER, Cook GA, et al. The early intervention referral process for rural infants and toddlers with delays or disabilities: a family perspective. Matern Child Health J 2021;25(5):715–23. https://doi.org/10.1007/s10995-020-03067-2.
76. Health Resources & Services Administration. The Maternal, Infant, and early Childhood Home Visiting program. Available at: https://mchb.hrsa.gov/sites/default/files/mchb/about-us/program-brief.pdf. Accessed February 14, 2024.
77. Brimsek E, Murdoch J, Chakraborti N. Exploring Remaining Needs and Opportunities for Improvement in Rural Communities: A Focus on Maternal, Infant, and Early Childhood Home Visiting (MIECHV) Services. OPRE Brief #2023-045. In: Office of Planning, Research, and Evaluation, Administration for Children and Families. Washington, DC: U.S. Department of Health and Human Services; 2022.
78. Jilani SM. Evaluation of state-mandated reporting of neonatal abstinence syndrome — six states, 2013–2017. MMWR Morb Mortal Wkly Rep 2019;68. https://doi.org/10.15585/mmwr.mm6801a2.
79. Warren MD, Miller AM, Traylor J, et al. Implementation of a statewide surveillance system for neonatal abstinence syndrome — Tennessee, 2013. Morb Mortal Wkly Rep 2015;64(5):125–8.
80. Umer A, Loudin S, Maxwell S, et al. Capturing the statewide incidence of neonatal abstinence syndrome in real time: the West Virginia experience. Pediatr Res 2019;85(5):607–11. https://doi.org/10.1038/s41390-018-0172-z.
81. Raphael JL, Wong SL. Addressing rural health disparities in neonatal abstinence syndrome: population-based surveillance and public policy. Pediatr Res 2019; 85(5):587–9. https://doi.org/10.1038/s41390-018-0272-9.

Optimizing the Care of Pediatric Injuries in Rural Environments

Kenneth W. Gow, MD[a], Mary E. Fallat, MD[b], Jonathan E. Kohler, MD[c,*]

KEYWORDS

• Pediatric • Injury • Trauma • Rural • Pediatric readiness

KEY POINTS

- Children in rural America have unique health care needs and face unique health care challenges related to increased risk of injury and decreased access to pediatric specialty care.
- Physicians in rural areas need to be prepared to care for children when pediatric specialty centers are not available or accessible.
- Numerous programs and standards exist to guide rural clinicians in developing high-quality pediatric readiness programs.

CASE STUDY

During the late evening of Friday, December 10, 2021, a violent, long-tracked EF4 tornado moved across Western Kentucky, causing catastrophic damage to numerous towns, including Mayfield, Princeton, Dawson Springs, and Bremen. There were estimated peak winds of 190 mph and a path length of 128 miles. The tornado was on the ground for 2 hours. Of the 78 fatalities, 12 were children. The affected area was rural, with the closest trauma center a Level IV that had lost both phone and Internet service. Helicopters could not fly. There were 22 injured children who were either triaged and transferred to more distant trauma centers or were treated and released at local hospitals. Of the children who made it to the hospital, all but one patient survived. Thankfully, such tragic disasters are rare. Still, rural pediatricians must be prepared to assist

[a] Division of Pediatric Surgery, Stony Brook University Hospital, 101 Nicolls Road, Stony Brook, NY 11794, USA; [b] The Hiram C. Polk, Jr., Department of Surgery, University of Louisville School of Medicine, Norton Children's Hospital, 315 East Broadway, Suite 565, Louisville, KY 40202, USA; [c] Division of Pediatric General, Thoracic and Fetal Surgery, University of California - Davis, 2335 Stockton Boulevard, 5th Floor, Sacramento, CA 95817, USA
* Corresponding author. 2335 Stockton Boulevard, 5th Floor, Sacramento, CA 95817.
E-mail address: jekohler@ucdavis.edu
Twitter: @MaryFallat (M.E.F.)

Pediatr Clin N Am 72 (2025) 53–63
https://doi.org/10.1016/j.pcl.2024.07.031 pediatric.theclinics.com
0031-3955/25/

injured patients until they can be stabilized or transferred to higher levels of care. As you read this article, consider the following questions:

1. As a pediatrician, are you aware of where the nearest trauma center is and whether it is "pediatric ready" and capable of taking care of an injured child?
2. What injury prevention initiatives do you ask about or provide education for in your office?
3. What is the role of the pediatrician in preparation and planning for a disaster involving children in their own community?
4. Do you know who your community partners are in planning and integration of children into all phases of emergency care where you live?

INTRODUCTION

Nearly 12 million children live in the rural United States.[1] Pediatric surgical care in rural environments presents unique challenges due to factors such as limited access to health care resources, long transport times to medical facilities, and disparities in emergency response infrastructure.[2] Common types of pediatric injuries in rural areas include those related to agriculture, recreational activities, motor vehicle accidents, and environmental hazards.[3] Studies indicate that rural children are at 55% higher risk of overall injury, double the risk of motor vehicle crash injury, 49% higher rate of unintentional drowning, and 47% higher suicide than urban children.[2,4] Addressing the increased risk of injury to rural children can be done through advocacy and prevention initiatives as these types of injuries all have potentially severe consequences to children's health and well-being. Preventive measures such as community education, safety training, and implementation of injury prevention programs tailored to the rural context are crucial for mitigating risks and promoting child safety.[2] Prompt access to appropriate medical care and trauma services is essential for reducing morbidity and mortality associated with pediatric injuries in rural settings. By recognizing the unique challenges of rural pediatric surgical care and implementing targeted interventions, health care providers, policymakers, and community stakeholders can work together to improve outcomes and reduce the burden of pediatric injuries in rural environments.[5] This article provides a brief review of pediatric rural injuries, what makes them unique, steps to minimize the frequency, and ways the current health care infrastructure can be improved to achieve better outcomes.[4] Integrating children's interests into all aspects of preparedness training makes the most sense such that taking care of children creates less apprehension on the part of the clinician.

UNDERSTANDING THE LANDSCAPE OF RURAL ENVIRONMENTS

The rural environment is characterized by vast geographic areas with sparse population density, limited access to health care facilities, and diverse socioeconomic backgrounds. These factors contribute to unique challenges in addressing pediatric injuries in rural settings. Limited availability of emergency medical services and trauma centers, coupled with long transport times to reach specialized care, can result in delays in treatment and worsen injury outcomes.[6] The prevalence of agricultural activities, outdoor recreational pursuits, and transportation-related risks in rural areas poses specific injury hazards to children.[3] Environmental factors such as rugged terrain, natural disasters, and exposure to wildlife contribute to the complexity of pediatric injury prevention and management in rural environments.[7] Socioeconomic disparities, including limited access to resources, education, preventive health care services, and primary care physicians, can exacerbate the vulnerability of rural children to injuries.[8] While 20% of American children live in rural communities, only 9% of general pediatricians or nurse practitioners practice in those areas.[9] Child poverty rates are higher in rural areas with nearly 1 in 4 rural children growing up in poverty.[10] These factors contribute to injury rates as much as 55% higher[2] and unintentional injury death rates twice that seen in urban settings for children who live in rural areas.[11] Addressing these challenges requires a multifaceted approach that encompasses community-based interventions, education, policy advocacy, and collaboration among health care providers, policymakers, and community stakeholders to mitigate the impact of pediatric injuries in rural settings.[4]

COMMON PEDIATRIC INJURIES IN RURAL ENVIRONMENTS

Common pediatric injuries in rural environments encompass a range of diverse hazards inherent to rural living. Agricultural-related injuries,[3] such as those sustained from farm machinery, livestock interactions, and falls from heights, are prevalent as many children help out on family farms in rural areas.[12] Farm injuries most commonly occur among youth ages from 15 to 19 years and are usually associated with the operation of heavy machinery. Many of these injured adolescents will require hospitalization.[13] The National Ag Safety Database indicates that agriculture is one of the most dangerous occupations in the country where children of any age can be present. Five sobering statistics include (1) a child dies in an agriculture-related incident every 3 days; (2) the number of agriculture-related youth workers is higher than all other industries combined; (3) many agriculture work-related injuries and deaths are associated with children doing work that does not match their developmental level; (4) 60% of child agriculture-related injuries happen to children who are not working; and (5) everyday, about 33 children are injured in an agriculture-related incident.[14] Outdoor recreational pursuits, including all terrain vehicle (ATV) riding,[12] biking, and hunting, also contribute to a notable proportion of pediatric injuries, often resulting from collisions, falls, or accidents involving firearms.[15,16] Motor vehicle accidents are a significant concern in rural settings, exacerbated by long stretches of highways, off roads in poor condition, and limited access to emergency medical services. Hung and colleagues[9] cite that vehicle crashes are more likely to be fatal in rural counties due to higher speeds, lower quality road design, and greater distances to hospitals. Emergency medical services may be voluntary and personnel less well trained to take care of injured children. Also, rural communities have lower levels of injury prevention behavior, such as seatbelt use, water safety practices, and use of bike helmets.[9] Environmental factors such as natural disasters, exposure to extreme weather conditions, and encounters with wildlife[17] pose risks to pediatric safety that are higher in rural environments. Overall, the diverse array of hazards present in rural areas underscores the importance of comprehensive injury prevention strategies tailored to address the specific challenges of pediatric safety in these settings. Pediatricians can access prevention tip sheets and information for parents through several organizations including the American Academy of Pediatrics (AAP) (The Injury Prevention Program [TIPP]),[18] SafeKids,[19] and 4-H.[20] Pediatric patient handouts from TIPP help pediatricians implement injury prevention counseling for parents of children newborn through aged 12 years for motor vehicles, firearms, bicycle crashes, drowning, poisoning, choking, burns, falls, and pedestrian hazards. SafeKids provides fact sheets on a number of injuries experienced by all ages of children and advice on prevention strategies for teachers, counselors, and parents. 4-H has more programs geared toward adolescents and promotes mentoring and provides strategies for coping with mental health challenges.

TRANSLATING "PREPARATION MEETS EMERGENCY" INTO EVERYDAY CARE

In 2020, the US census data were updated and many of the statistics that give guidance to rural America are updated more frequently on the Rural Health Information Hub.[21] The US population in 2022 was estimated at 333 million.[22] Rural Americans reside in 72% of the total United States land area but only comprise 14% of the population (46 million).[23]

Nearly a quarter (22.2%) of those living in rural areas as of 2021 are children aged less than 18 years (13.4 million). Overall, 11.6% of families live in poverty and approximately 19 million Americans (6% of the population) still lack access to fixed broadband service at threshold speeds, which has implications for promulgating telehealth as a strategy for patient care. In rural areas, nearly 25% of the population (14.5 million people) lack access to this service. **Fig. 1** depicts the current status of rurality by state based on the last census.[24]

Access to trauma care for children who live in rural and underserved areas can be challenging because of access to primary care, emergency care, workforce capable of caring for children, and insurance plans that may dictate referral patterns. Access to care can also be greatly affected by geography, weather, and transportation with the latter 2 situational and codependent on availability of transport over a distance to tertiary care.

In 2022, according to the American Hospital Association (AHA) Annual Survey database, there were 6093 US hospitals, of which 5139 were considered community hospitals and 1796 of these were considered rural community hospitals. At the same time, there were approximately 279 children's hospitals. An article published in 2020 intentionally tried to discriminate children's hospitals from non-children's hospitals using an American Hospital Association Healthcare Institute Claims database from 2015.[25] There were 4464 hospitals in the database and they were tiered according to pediatric services. There were 5 tiers with Tier A being freestanding children's hospitals (51), B having key pediatric services and characterized by children's hospitals within a larger hospital or system (228), C having limited pediatric services (1721), D having no

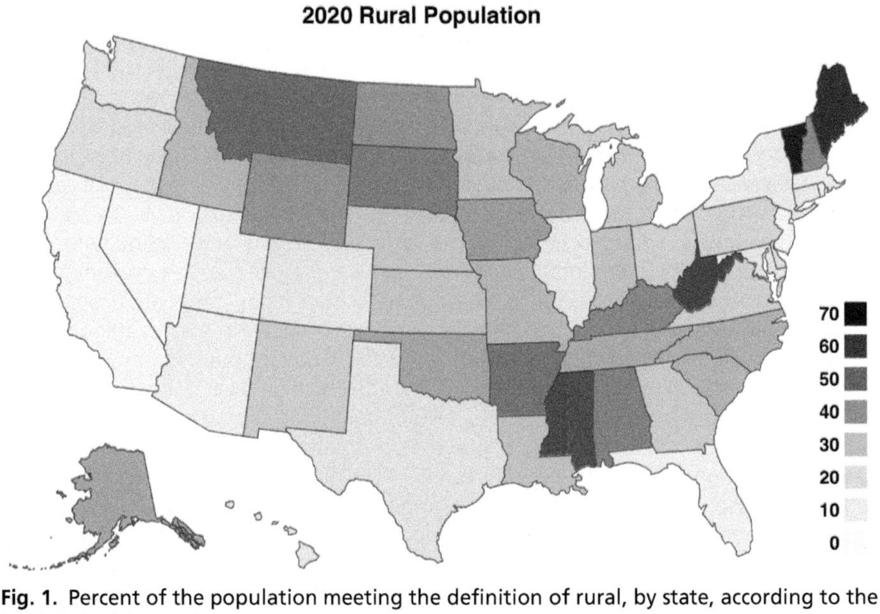

Fig. 1. Percent of the population meeting the definition of rural, by state, according to the 2020 United States Census.

pediatric services (1728), and E unclassified (738). According to claims data, the percentage of admissions that were pediatric was highest in tier A (88.9%), followed by tiers B (10.9%), C (3.9%), and D (3.9%). Of interest, 28.06% of admissions at unclassified hospitals were pediatric, although the services provided were not robust. Pertinent is the number of states in the northern plains and midwest where the number of children's hospitals is far fewer. In 2020, Fallat and colleagues[26] studied pediatric trauma system development and integration across the country. Each state was assigned a score based on 6 domains of planning and development that affect children's care: disaster, legislation, and funding; access to care; injury prevention and recognition; quality improvement and trauma registry; and pediatric readiness. The entire report is available as a PDF download and is accessible on the Emergency Medical Services for Children (EMSC) Innovation and Improvement Center (EIIC) Web site.[27] The maximum score was 100, but the study showed that many states lack a number of essential resources for children. A blueprint for helping states improve their resources for children has recently been published.[28]

STRATEGIES FOR INTERVENTION: PEDIATRIC READINESS COMES OF AGE FOR TRAUMA CENTERS

Being "ready," willing or capable of performing a task has taken on new meaning since the stresses to the health care system associated with the corona virus disease of 2019 (COVID-19) pandemic. "Readiness" as defined as "being fully prepared for something" is now much more about being ready everyday for the mass casualty event that might take place tomorrow. It used to be easier for a trauma or acute care surgery team to say, "we do not take care of kids here" and to send the children to a center that specializes in pediatric care. As we consider the consequences and increasing frequency of mass shootings and of climate change and natural disasters (tornados, hurricanes, floods, mudslides, fires, and the threat of earthquakes), there will be circumstances where children must be managed in a rural or underserved environment at least temporarily and possibly for days until a tertiary or quaternary center can accept them in transfer. High-level pediatric trauma centers are also at risk to be damaged or inaccessible during a disaster.

The American College of Surgeons Committee on Trauma has partnered with the programs in the Health Resources and Services Administration (HRSA) including the EMSC and the EIIC to promote the importance of "pediatric readiness" in the emergency departments of trauma centers and Emergency Medical Services (EMS) Services.[29,30] There are several other key stakeholders in pediatric readiness, including the AAP, the American College of Emergency Physicians, and the Society for Trauma Nurses. Two recent publications highlighted the survival benefits of a pediatric-ready emergency department for ill and injured children,[31,32] but it also makes sense that injured patients of any age should be taken to a higher level pediatric trauma center preferentially. There are many areas of the country, particularly in the northern plains and western parts of the United States where pediatric trauma centers are hours away from injured children and children need to be triaged to and stabilized at adult-centered hospitals, some of which see few children in their emergency departments daily. The pediatric readiness project enables the emergency department team to better prepare for medical and surgical emergencies that involve children. A standardized checklist helps the emergency department (ED) team understand the gaps in equipment, supplies, medications and dosing, education, training, protocols, and transfer agreements needed to optimize care.[33] The program also champions designation of a key person or pediatric emergency care coordinator (PECC) to be the program manager in charge of pediatric readiness. Optimally, there will be a physician and nurse dyad who can oversee quality improvement and make sure there are quality and safety programs in place.

Beginning in August 2023 when the new resources for optimal care of the injured patient ("The Gray Book") went into effect, the American College of Surgeons trauma center verification program now has a pediatric readiness standard in place for all levels of trauma center verified by the American College of Surgeons (ACS) (**Table 1**).[34] The best way to approach the standard is to work with a hospital's emergency department team, who will oversee making sure your local trauma center or hospital is pediatric ready (**Box 1**). Responsibilities for trauma centers will include understanding gaps in care for children and having a plan in place to address the gaps, but this should be the goal for all hospitals.

Standard 5.10—Pediatric Readiness

Understanding that pediatric readiness in rural and underserved areas of the country is still in evolution, what does good look like in a rural environment with respect to children's injury and disaster care, where many clinicians will see few children in practice? The answer to this question is dependent on many factors. These include training various levels of clinician to provide emergency care, including physicians, nurses, respiratory therapy, radiology technicians, and emergency medical services. If there are pediatric inpatient services at any level, there must be an infrastructure to support them, including physicians and nurses with the skill set needed for the hospital scope of services. The technology must support children, which requires administrative buy in. The public must have confidence in their local hospital and providers, at least for front-line services. Participation in quality improvement is also paramount to the successful care of children.

The best model on which to build an infrastructure for children's services in a rural setting begins with building a network of care with bidirectional communication between a children's hospital and the rural hospital. This communication may allow some children to safely stay at home but will also facilitate the stabilization and safe transport of children who need to be moved to a higher level of care. Having established protocols and procedures in place is essential to make this transition of care as smooth as possible. But this is not enough. Children must be integrated into every aspect of state planning and preparedness to ensure that their needs can be

Table 1
American College of Surgeons standard for pediatric readiness, now applicable to every level of trauma center verification[34]

Applicable Levels	LI, LII, LIII, PTCI, PTCII
Definition and Requirements	In all trauma centers, the emergency department must evaluate its pediatric readiness and have a plan to address any deficiencies.
Additional Information	"Pediatric readiness" refers to infrastructure, administration and coordination of care, personnel, pediatric-specific policies, equipment, and other resources that ensure the center is prepared to provide care to an injured child. The components that define readiness are available in the resources link in the following. https://emscimprovement.center/domains/pediatric-readiness-project/readiness-toolkit/
Measures of Compliance	Gap analysis with plan to address deficiencies in pediatric readiness

Box 1
Opportunities for better preparation of hospitals to care for kids everyday and in disaster planning

1. Have a "pediatric-ready" emergency department
2. Have at least one PECC for your local ED and EMS service and Trauma Program if you have one
3. Develop transfer guidelines and protocols for a higher level of care with agreements in place
4. Pediatric Advanced Life Support (PALS) versus Advanced Trauma Life Support (ATLS) or both for the "front-line" emergency care providers
5. As low as reasonably achievable guidelines to minimize exposure to ionizing radiation and minimize workup to the essential needs
6. Use national evidence-based pediatric protocols such as those developed through the Pediatric Emergency Care Applied Research Network (https://pecarn.org) or the EIIC (https://emscimprovement.center)
7. Consider using telehealth as a bridge to definitive care
8. Make sure children are considered in your hospital disaster plan including surge capacity
9. Affiliate with your State EMSC (https://mchb.hrsa.gov/programs-impact/emergency-medical-services-children-emsc)

Program Director and Manager to understand how your hospital ED can improve care for all kids

10. Coordinate your hospital's preparedness plans with your State Emergency Management and State Hospital Preparedness Program to make sure children are integrated into the state plan
11. Coordinate with your State Committee on Trauma Chair to make sure children are integrated into your State Trauma Plan and someone with children's expertise is on the Trauma Advisory Council

addressed not only everyday but in a disaster. This includes relationship building by hospitals with State partners such as emergency management, the State Hospital Association and Hospital Preparedness Programs, EMS for Children and the State EMS agency, the State Department for Public Health, and the State Trauma System. All of these entities must come together in a disaster and children must be considered in the planning phase. In some states, there are already more sophisticated Medical Operations Control Centers (MOCCs) and integration of children's interests going forward will be designated as Pediatric Medical Operations Control Centers (P-MOCC). This is a goal for every State. The HRSA funds EMSC, the EIIC, and now the Pediatric Pandemic Network, a network of 10 children's hospital hubs and associated infrastructure to develop a national all-hazards approach to disasters in children.[35] The Administration for Strategic Preparedness and Response at the US Department of Health and Human Services has several Disaster Centers of Excellence that regionally address disaster preparedness.[36] Alignment of your local hospital with any of these efforts will go a long way to guaranteeing that the children in your community receive better care, both everyday and in the event of a disaster.

FUTURE DIRECTIONS AND RECOMMENDATIONS

Clinicians who care for patients in rural areas face unique challenges in caring for a varied population with a wide variety of needs in a resource-limited setting. One of the most limited resources in rural pediatric care is basic knowledge about the population and the clinicians who serve them. Compared to urban academic medical centers, which often participate in large multicenter data and quality-sharing programs, rural medicine has very little centralized data, making research into the needs of rural hospitals and patients difficult. Basic questions, like what operations are performed on children in what setting, with what resources and by what types of physician, are essentially impossible to answer at a national scale with existing data sources. Improving data gathering and accessibility for rural pediatric surgical care is essential to developing policies and programs to effectively support high-quality care of rural children.

There are multiple programs working to improve the surgical care of rural children by creating resources for pediatric readiness and networks of pediatric specialists eager to engage with rural partners to develop the sorts of data and quality programs that are necessary for high-quality pediatric care. National programs such as the Pediatric Pandemic Network and the Pediatric Readiness Project have been joined by regional programs such as the Western Regional Alliance for Pediatric Emergency Management[37] to create layers of pediatric specialist support for rural providers. While some degree of pediatric readiness can be mandated by programs such as the American College of Surgeons trauma verification program, the most essential component for developing high-quality rural pediatric surgical care is the interest and enthusiasm of rural clinicians and the facilities where they work. These programs cannot be effective without engagement by, and leadership from, the rural providers they hope to serve.

There are exciting innovations in technology that may also help bring pediatric speciality care to rural environments. Although the COVID-19 pandemic placed unprecedented strain on rural health care systems, it also catalyzed a remarkable transformation in the accessibility and acceptability of telehealth systems to provide remote care. From video-based clinic visits to "telepresence" systems that allow specialists to remotely evaluate and treat patients over the Internet, technological solutions to getting specialists into rural areas have proliferated and regulatory and administrative barriers have lowered. Still, there will never be a substitute to "boots on the ground"—rural clinicians who are able, willing, and ready to care for the children in their own communities.

SUMMARY

Rural children are at a higher risk for injury at baseline and are uniquely at risk in disaster situations where access to prompt pediatric speciality care is not available or accessible. Though sparsely populated by definition, much of the United States land mass is rural, and millions of rural children depend on local clinicians to provide either definitive care or at least evaluation and stabilization before transfer to a pediatric center. Rural pediatric preparedness initiatives exist to promote high-quality local care for rural children, but these programs have largely been developed by large, urban, academic centers. To be truly successful, any rural preparedness program requires that rural clinicians engage and guide these programs to be most relevant and useful to the communities they serve.

CLINICS CARE POINTS

- Rural children have increased incidence of injury and a different injury pattern than urban children, though the differences between rural and urban pediatric care remain poorly understood.

- Injury prevention resources for rural children exist through multiple agencies including the AAP and SafeKids.
- Pediatric readiness is an essential component to rural pediatric care, and multiple resources exist to help hospitals and clinicians be "peds ready." Some, such as the Pediatric Readiness checklist, are now mandated for trauma center verification.
- A pediatric disaster plan is necessary for rural hospitals, but the best preparation for caring for children in a disaster is having systems in place to provide high-quality care for children under normal circumstances.

DISCLOSURE

The authors have nothing to disclose.

REFERENCES

1. Probst J, Zahnd W, Breneman C. Declines In Pediatric Mortality Fall Short For Rural US Children. Health Aff Proj Hope 2019;38(12):2069–76.
2. Ficker E. Health Disparities in Rural Childhood Injury | Children's Safety Network. Available at: https://www.childrenssafetynetwork.org/blog/health-disparities-rural-childhood-injury. [Accessed 26 February 2024].
3. Lee BC, Salzwedel MA. Safeguarding youth from agricultural injury and illness: The United States' experience. Front Public Health 2023;11:1048576.
4. Kim K, Ozegovic D, Voaklander DC. Differences in incidence of injury between rural and urban children in Canada and the USA: a systematic review. Inj Prev 2012;18(4):264–71.
5. Pai PK, Klinkner DB. Pediatric trauma in the rural and low resourced communities. Semin Pediatr Surg 2022;31(5):151222.
6. Warshaw R. Health Disparities Affect Millions in Rural U.S. Communities. AAMC. Available at: https://www.aamc.org/news/health-disparities-affect-millions-rural-us-communities. [Accessed 26 February 2024].
7. Bettenhausen JL, Winterer CM, Colvin JD. Health and Poverty of Rural Children: An Under-Researched and Under-Resourced Vulnerable Population. Acad Pediatr 2021;21(8):S126–33.
8. Seshamani M, Jacobs D, Moody-Williams J, et al. Addressing Rural Health Inequities in Medicare, Available at: https://www.cms.gov/blog/addressing-rural-health-inequities-medicare. (Accessed 26 February 2024).
9. Hung P, Workman M, Mohan K. NRHA Policy Paper: Overview of Rural Child Health. Published online 2020. Accessed February 26, 2024. Available at: https://www.ruralhealth.us/NRHA/media/Emerge_NRHA/Advocacy/Policy%20documents/2020-NRHA-Policy-Document-Overview-of-Rural-Child-Health.pdf.
10. t. Growing Up in Rural America: U.S. complement to the End of Childhood report 2018. Save the Children's Resource Centre. Available at: https://resourcecentre.savethechildren.net/pdf/2018-end-of-childhood-report-us.pdf/. [Accessed 26 February 2024].
11. Garnett MF, Spencer MR, Hedegaard H. Urban-rural Differences in Unintentional Injury Death Rates Among Children Aged 0-17 Years: United States, 2018-2019. NCHS Data Brief 2021;421:1–8.
12. VanWormer JJ, Berg RL, Burke RR, et al. Regional surveillance of medically-attended farm-related injuries in children and adolescents. Front Public Health 2022;10:1031618.

13. Zagel AL, Kreykes NS, Handt EA. Pediatric Farm Injuries Presenting to United States Emergency Departments, 2001-2014. J Rural Health 2019;35(4):442–52.
14. NASD - National Children's Center for Rural and Agricultural Health and Safety (NCCRAHS). Available at: http://nasdonline.org. [Accessed 26 February 2024].
15. Kaufman EJ, Wiebe DJ, Xiong RA, et al. Epidemiologic Trends in Fatal and Nonfatal Firearm Injuries in the US, 2009-2017. JAMA Intern Med 2021; 181(2):237.
16. Herrin BR, Gaither JR, Leventhal JM, et al. Rural Versus Urban Hospitalizations for Firearm Injuries in Children and Adolescents. Pediatrics 2018;142(2): e20173318.
17. Massand S, Giglio M, Patel A, et al. Uncovering a Failed Pediatric Patient Population in Rural America: A Statewide Analysis of Over 1,000 Dog Bite Injuries. Cureus 2022. https://doi.org/10.7759/cureus.25734.
18. American Academy of Pediatrics. TIPP (The Injury Prevention Program). TIPP (The Injury Prevention Program). Available at: https://publications.aap.org/patiented/pages/c_tipp?autologincheck=redirected. [Accessed 5 March 2024].
19. Safety Tips. Safe Kids Worldwide. Available at: https://www.safekids.org/safetytips. [Accessed 5 March 2024].
20. About 4H. National 4-H Council. Available at: https://4-h.org/about/. [Accessed 9 March 2024].
21. Rural Health Information Hub. Available at: https://www.ruralhealthinfo.org/. [Accessed 5 March 2024].
22. U.S. Census Bureau QuickFacts: United States. Available at: https://www.census.gov/quickfacts/fact/table/US/PST045222. [Accessed 2 March 2024].
23. Ratcliffe M, Burd C, Holder K, et al. Defining Rural at the U.S. Census Bureau. Available at: https://www.census.gov/library/publications/2016/acs/acsgeo-1.html.
24. Most Rural States 2024. Available at: https://worldpopulationreview.com/state-rankings/most-rural-states. [Accessed 2 March 2024].
25. Piper KN, Baxter KJ, McCarthy I, et al. Distinguishing Children's Hospitals From Non-Children's Hospitals in Large Claims Data. Hosp Pediatr 2020;10(2):123–8.
26. Fallat ME, Treager C, Humphrey S, et al. A Novel Approach to Assessment of US Pediatric Trauma System Development. JAMA Surg 2022;157(11):1042.
27. Fallat ME, Collings AT. Pediatric Trauma System Development In The United States. Available at: https://media.emscimprovement.center/documents/202302-Report-Digital-PTSAS.pdf. [Accessed 5 March 2024].
28. Stephens CQ, Fallat ME. Setting an agenda for a national pediatric trauma system: Operationalization of the Pediatric Trauma State Assessment Score. J Trauma Acute Care Surg 2023. https://doi.org/10.1097/TA.0000000000004208.
29. Ross SW, Campion E, Jensen AR, et al. Prehospital and emergency department pediatric readiness for injured children: A statement from the American College of Surgeons Committee on Trauma Emergency Medical Services Committee. J Trauma Acute Care Surg 2023;95(2):e6–10.
30. National Pediatric Readiness Project. Emergency Medical Services for Children Innovation and Improvement Center (EIIC). Available at: https://emscimprovement.center/domains/pediatric-readiness-project/. [Accessed 8 March 2024].
31. Ames SG, Davis BS, Marin JR, et al. Emergency Department Pediatric Readiness and Mortality in Critically Ill Children. Pediatrics 2019;144(3):e20190568.
32. Newgard CD, Lin A, Malveau S, et al. Emergency Department Pediatric Readiness and Short-term and Long-term Mortality Among Children Receiving Emergency Care. JAMA Netw Open 2023;6(1):e2250941.

33. Pediatric Readiness Assessment - Home Page. Available at: https://www.pedsready.org/. [Accessed 8 March 2024].
34. Resources for Optimal Care of the Injured Patient. ACS. Available at: https://www.facs.org/quality-programs/trauma/quality/verification-review-and-consultation-program/standards/. [Accessed 8 March 2024].
35. Pediatric Pandemic Network. Available at: https://pedspandemicnetwork.org/. [Accessed 8 March 2024].
36. ASPR | Homepage. Available at: https://aspr.hhs.gov:443/Pages/Home.aspx. [Accessed 8 March 2024].
37. WRAP-EM. Western Regional Alliance for Pediatric Emergency Management (WRAP-EM). Accessed. Available at: https://www.wrap-em.org/. [Accessed 8 March 2024].

A Call for Pediatric Clinicians to Address Environmental Health Concerns in Rural Settings

Rachel Criswell, MD, MS[a,b,c,*], Kelsey Gleason, ScD, MS[d], Ahlam K. Abuawad, PhD[b], Margaret R. Karagas, PhD[b], Kathleen Grene, MD, MPH[e], Ana M. Mora, MD, PhD[f], Brenda Eskenazi, MA, PhD[f], Katie Senechal, SM[g,h], Anne M. Mullin, BS[c], Lisa B. Rokoff, PhD[c,h], Abby F. Fleisch, MD, MPH[c,h,i]

KEYWORDS

• Wood stove • Well water • Biosolids • Pesticides • Environmental health • Rural health

Continued

INTRODUCTION

Rural populations encounter a unique set of environmental hazards. With fewer people and more space, public infrastructure tends to be sparse or nonexistent. Thus, residents rely more heavily on local resources, such as wood stoves for heating and private wells for water. Wood stoves emit air pollutants that lower indoor air quality, and private wells, often untested, frequently carry contaminants. Additionally, agriculture remains one of the primary industries of the rural United States,[1] bringing with it

[a] Skowhegan Family Medicine, Redington-Fairview General Hospital, 46 Fairview Avenue, Suite 334, PO Box 468, Skowhegan, ME 04976, USA; [b] Department of Epidemiology, Geisel School of Medicine and Children's Environmental Health and Disease Prevention Research Center at Dartmouth, 1 Medical Center Drive, Williamson Building, 7th Floor, Lebanon, NH 03756, USA; [c] Tufts University School of Medicine, 136 Harrison Avenue, Boston, MA 02111, USA; [d] Department of Biomedical and Health Sciences, University of Vermont, 106 Carrigan Drive, Rowell Building, Burlington, VT 05405, USA; [e] Pediatrics, Yale-New Haven Hospital, New Haven, CT, USA; [f] Center for Environmental Research and Community Health (CERCH), School of Public Health, University of California, 1995 University Avenue, Suite 265, Berkeley, CA 94704, USA; [g] Department of Epidemiology, Harvard T.H. Chan School of Public Health, 677 Huntington Avenue, Boston, MA 02115, USA; [h] Center for Interdisciplinary and Population Health Research, MaineHealth Institute for Research, 1 Riverfront Plaza, Floor 4, Westbrook, ME 04902, USA; [i] Pediatric Endocrinology and Diabetes, Maine Medical Center, 887 Congress Street, Suite 300, Portland, ME 04102, USA
* Corresponding author. Skowhegan Family Medicine, Redington-Fairview General Hospital, 46 Fairview Avenue, Suite 334, Skowhegan, ME 04976.
E-mail address: rcriswell@rfgh.net

Pediatr Clin N Am 72 (2025) 65–83
https://doi.org/10.1016/j.pcl.2024.07.030 pediatric.theclinics.com

Continued

KEY POINTS

- Children in rural settings are exposed to environmental hazards including air pollution from wood stoves, well water contaminants, and agricultural exposures such as biosolids and pesticides.
- Compared to adults, children experience a closer interaction with the environment, and their developing physiology places them at risk for long-term health effects from contaminants such as particulate matter, heavy metals, perfluoroalkyl and polyfluoroalkyl substances, and pesticides.
- Pediatric clinicians can use existing tools to screen for environmental health risks and support families through mitigation, testing, and medical monitoring.

pollutants associated with biosolids (treated sewage used as fertilizer) and pesticides. Recent articles have highlighted the necessity of including rural populations in an environmental justice framework.[2–4]

Children are particularly susceptible to environmental exposures because they consume, breathe, and ingest more on a per-kilogram basis than adults,[5] have a physiologically thinner dermal barrier,[6–8] and have less mature metabolisms and immune systems to counteract harmful exposures.[9] Further, children participate in more hand-to-mouth activity, have less autonomy in decision-making regarding exposures, and have unique exposure routes such as via human milk.[10,11] Once exposures have occurred, children also have longer subsequent lifespans during which health effects may occur, and exposures during early life and other key developmental periods may have "programming" effects that can affect health well into adulthood.[12]

In this targeted review, the authors describe 3 environmental hazards in rural settings: (1) wood stove smoke, (2) well water contaminants, and (3) agricultural pollutants including biosolids and pesticides. They detail the prevalence of these exposures and evidence linking these exposures with adverse health outcomes, thereby emphasizing their considerable public health importance (**Fig. 1**). They also describe how climate change may exacerbate these exposures and how these environmental hazards unique to rural life may magnify preexisting health disparities between children living in rural areas and those living in urban areas.

Surveys of medical education curricula and clinician perceptions of self-efficacy indicate that counseling regarding environmental health exposures is an area of growth for most practicing clinicians.[13] The authors encourage clinicians seeing patients living in rural areas to screen for these exposures, and they provide concrete evidence, advice, and resources for clinicians to help vulnerable and affected patients mitigate exposures.

DISCUSSION

Wood Stove Smoke

Prevalence of wood stove use

In the United States, wood is the primary heating fuel for 2.25 million households and a secondary source of heating for nearly 9 million households.[14] Residential wood stove use is highest in New England and the Mountain North regions,[14] with individuals living in rural states with high forest covers such as Vermont (13.1%), Maine (8.6%), and Montana (6.5%)[15,16] reporting the greatest use of wood stoves as their primary household heat source per the 2022 US Census[17] (**Fig. 2**).

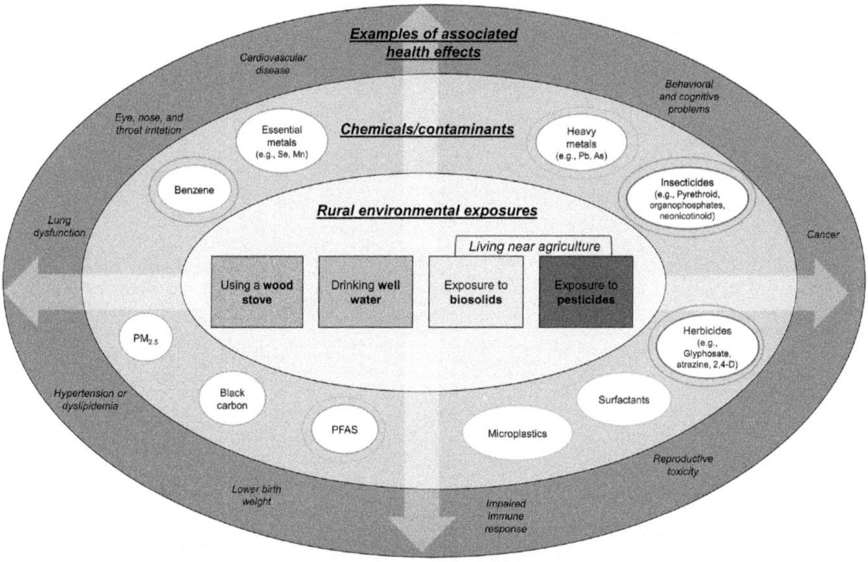

Fig. 1. Rural environmental exposures, associated color-coded chemicals/contaminants (from using a wood stove [*orange*], drinking well water [*blue*], exposure to biosolids [*light green*], and exposure to pesticides [*dark green*]), and examples of associated adverse health effects.

Contaminants in wood stove smoke

Wood stove smoke contains a heterogeneous mixture of gaseous and particulate air pollutants resulting from the incomplete combustion of burned firewood.[6] Wood smoke is primarily composed of particulate matter that is 2.5 μm or smaller in diameter ($PM_{2.5}$). When inhaled, $PM_{2.5}$ reaches deep into the alveoli and distal airways of the lungs.[18] Wood stove smoke also contains other pollutants including trace elements, carbon monoxide, polycyclic aromatic hydrocarbons, and formaldehyde, among others (**Box 1**).[19,20]

In northern New England, black carbon, a toxic component of $PM_{2.5}$, is on average 62% higher in homes with versus without a wood stove. Black carbon is known to be a major pollutant in automobile exhaust,[21] yet concentrations of black carbon in homes with a wood stove in northern New England were higher than levels reported in homes in nearby urban Boston, Massachusetts.[20] Wood stoves are used primarily during winter months when children spend more time indoors, increasing exposure potential.

Health effects of wood stove smoke exposure

Reduced indoor air quality from wood stove smoke impacts an estimated 3 million children in the United States.[6,22] Robust evidence links $PM_{2.5}$ and black carbon exposure with respiratory outcomes such as wheezing and asthma during childhood.[23] Greater black carbon exposure has also been associated with adverse cardiovascular health and premature mortality among children and adults.[21] A recent study identified an association between wood stove use and incident lung cancer, adding evidence to the International Agency for Research on Cancer's (IARC) characterization of indoor emissions from wood fuel as "probably carcinogenic" to humans.[24,25] Studies have also found that pregnant people exposed to wood stove smoke are more likely to have abnormal glycemia during pregnancy and small-for-gestational-age infants.[26]

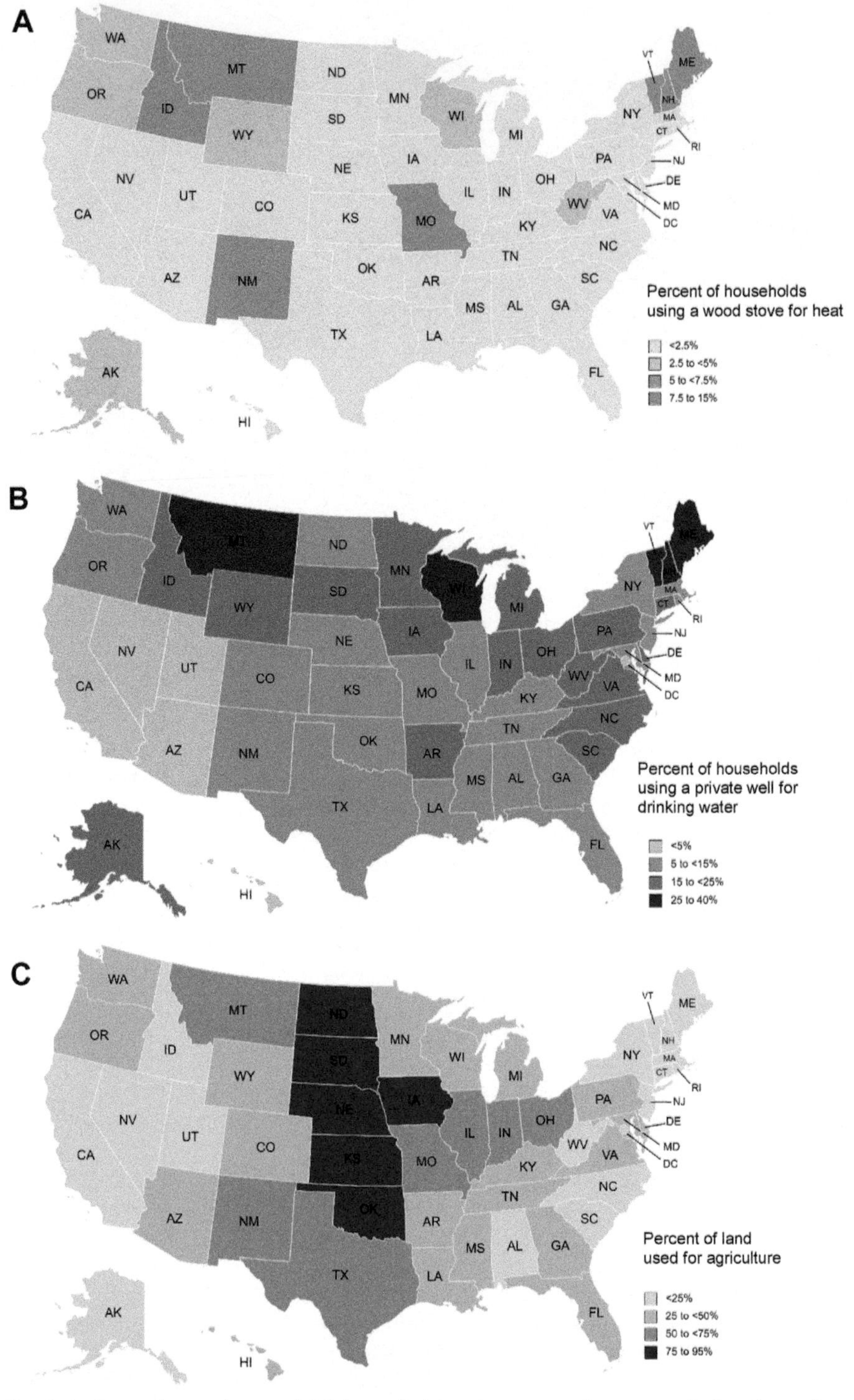

Fig. 2. Estimated prevalence of (*A*) households using a wood stove as their primary heat source, (*B*) households using a private well for drinking water, and (*C*) land used for agriculture, for the 50 states in the United States.[17,29,56,57]

Box 1
Examples of air pollutants common in smoke from wood stoves

Black carbon
- Elemental carbon
- Organic carbon
- Potassium
- Trace elements (eg, calcium, selenium, chlorine, sulfur)
- Carbon monoxide
- Polycyclic aromatic hydrocarbons
- Toxic organic compounds (eg, benzene, 1,3 butadiene, benzo[α]pyrene)
- Nitrogen oxides
- Formaldehyde

The particles present in smoke from wood stoves are categorized by their size. Smoke from wood stoves is primarily composed of particulate matter that is 2.5 μm or smaller in diameter ($PM_{2.5}$), and many of the pollutants listed here are present in $PM_{2.5}$.

Well Water

Prevalence of private wells

The US Environmental Protection Agency (EPA) estimated that more than 23 million US households acquired drinking water from private wells in 2010.[27] Private wells are most prevalent in rural regions where access to municipal or public water utilities is unavailable. Areas with the highest density of private well use (>90 people/km^2) are in the Northeast, around the Great Lakes and Southwest, and in areas scattered across the remaining United States (see **Fig. 2**).[28,29]

Public policies around well water testing

Although guidelines exist, most states do not regulate private well maintenance and testing. This stems from the 1974 Safe Drinking Water Act, which limits state and federal regulations to water systems with greater than 15 service connections or serving greater than 25 people, excluding Native American reservations. Thus, the onus falls on the homeowner to test their private well water to ensure it is safe for drinking. Many homeowners may not be aware of guidelines,[30] despite recommendations by state health departments and other organizations such as the American Academy of Pediatrics (AAP).[31] Data on the prevalence of private well testing are scant, but studies from New Jersey, Wisconsin, and New Hampshire indicate that few homeowners test their wells in accordance with guidelines, even when state testing regulations exist.[32–34]

Contaminants in well water

Private well water contaminants depend on multiple factors including well depth and type (ie, dug versus drilled), geologic landscape, type of aquifer, and anthropogenic sources of contamination (eg, local industrial practices and land use). We list common contaminants in **Box 2**.[31,35,36] Contaminants can be introduced into private wells through multiple sources, but industrial processes that produce surface water runoff/seepage and move into groundwater are a common pathway. For example, nitrates/nitrites, naturally occurring nitrogen-based molecules that can be harmful when consumed in excess, may be introduced into private wells via sewage, fertilizer, or animal waste. Sewage and animal waste are likewise pathways for pharmaceuticals to enter private wells. Industrial waste and plumbing/service lines can also leach contaminants into household water supplies.[28] Perfluoroalkyl and polyfluoroalkyl substances (PFAS), endocrine-disrupting chemicals added to nonstick and oil-resistant

Box 2
Common contaminants in well water

Nitrates/nitrites
- Heavy metals
- Essential metals (eg, selenium)
- Fluoride
- Radon gas
- PFAS
- Volatile organic compounds (eg, benzene)
- Pesticides
- Microorganisms
- Fracking chemicals (eg, benzene, formaldehyde, and chlorine)
- Disinfection byproducts (eg, trihalomethanes, haloacetic acids, chlorite, and bromate)
- Pharmaceuticals (eg, antimicrobials and hormones)

consumer products, and pesticides can be introduced via products used in agricultural or industrial practices. Disinfection byproducts (DBPs) may contaminate private wells in communities where water is improperly chlorinated.[36] Factors influencing contaminant levels include drought or flooding, proximity to industrial sites, and availability of testing and filtration systems. Well water contamination may also result in contamination of local food systems, with products such as locally produced eggs and produce and wild game and fish being further routes of exposure.[37]

Health effects of contaminated well water exposure

Aside from the pathogenic effects of microbial contaminants, substantial epidemiologic evidence links private well water contaminants to adverse health impacts. Heavy metals and essential elements such as arsenic, chromium VI, uranium, and radon have been deemed Group I human carcinogens by IARC,[38] while lead, selenium, and nitrates/nitrites are considered probable or possible human carcinogens.[39–41] Beyond carcinogenicity, short-term, high-dose exposure to uranium can result in kidney damage,[42] while long-term exposure to arsenic has been associated with increased risk of developing cardiovascular disease and diabetes.[43] Exposure to both arsenic and lead can interfere with neurodevelopment and growth.[44–48] Even exposure to essential elements at high levels can have toxic effects: for example, selenium has been associated with hypertension,[49] and exposure to manganese with perturbations in neurodevelopment and growth.[50–55] DBPs have been associated with reproductive toxicity.[36]

AGRICULTURAL EXPOSURES

Agriculture remains a steady industry and major source of employment in the rural United States (see **Fig. 2**).[1,56,57] Agriculture poses unique environmental hazards to children living on or near farmland, who may be exposed to biosolids and pesticides.

Biosolids

Prevalence of biosolids

Biosolids are semi-solid materials formed after human and industrial wastes are treated physically and chemically at wastewater treatment plants. In the United States, over 15,000 wastewater treatment plants need to dispose of biosolids.[58] Some biosolids are incinerated or put into landfills, but because of their high level of nitrogen, phosphorus, and organic carbon, over half of all biosolids are reused as fertilizer.[59,60] From 1998 to 2010, biosolids, referred to colloquially as "sludge," were applied to over 1.2 million acres of farmland annually in the United States. While on the decline, this practice has continued with over 800,000 acres impacted in 2018. Many fields have over 20 years of biosolids application with the highest application density in the eastern United States.[61,62]

Routes of childhood exposure to biosolids

Children are typically exposed to biosolids via drinking water contamination; biosolids used as fertilizer seep into the ground and groundwater, where they contaminate residential drinking wells.[63,64] Other suspected pathways of exposure include consuming crops or meat and dairy raised on feed grown in soil fertilized with biosolids and consuming wild game or fish living in biosolid-contaminated areas.[65]

Contaminants in biosolids

Biosolids used as fertilizer pose health risks because while the current sewage treatment process removes bacteria and other microorganisms, it cannot completely remove contaminants such as PFAS, microplastics, pharmaceuticals, surfactants, and heavy metals (**Box 3**).[66] These pollutants enter wastewater by being flushed down the toilet or excreted from the body via stool or urine. In addition, contaminants such as PFAS and microplastics in clothing and cleaning agents can enter wastewater from washing machines.[67] Other contaminants, particularly heavy metals, enter wastewater through stormwater runoff, especially in areas where sewer and stormwater collection systems are combined.[67]

Health effects of contaminated biosolids exposure

Each of the contaminants in biosolids has been independently associated with health risks. PFAS, which persist in the environment and have a long (3–8 year) biologic half-life in humans,[68,69] are associated with decreased antibody response to vaccines, dyslipidemia, increased kidney and testicular cancer risk, and lower birth weight.[63,70,71] The IARC has classified perfluorooctanoic acid as "carcinogenic to humans" and perfluorooctanesulfanoic acid as "possibly carcinogenic to humans."[72]

Microplastics, plastics less than 5000 μm in diameter, concentrate in the gastrointestinal tract, liver, kidney, and muscle and lead to oxidative stress, mitochondrial dysfunction, and inflammation, as well as metabolic toxicity and reproductive dysfunction in animal studies.[73–75] Population-based studies in humans have suggested possible associations with inflammatory bowel disease and lung injury.[73,76,77] While microplastics are ubiquitous, newer techniques that are able to detect nanoplastics (<1 μm in diameter) have indicated that the presence of these contaminants in drinking water is likely orders of magnitude higher than previously reported for microplastics alone.[78]

Pharmaceuticals such as antimicrobials and hormones are also found in biosolids, and exposure to these can promote the development of antibiotic-resistant bacteria and interfere with estrogen receptors and other reproductive and developmental pathways.[66,79–82]

Box 3
Common contaminants in biosolids that are not removed during sewage treatment

PFAS
Microplastics
Pharmaceuticals (eg, antimicrobials and hormones)
Surfactants
Heavy metals

Surfactants contain alkylphenol ethoxylates, a family of synthetic organic chemicals that accumulate in US biosolids in amounts that far exceed limits set for European countries.[83] Surfactants and their metabolites have endocrine-disrupting properties and have been associated with nervous system anomalies.[83,84]

Heavy metals are present in biosolids, and their concentrations are largely regulated by the US EPA Part 503 Biosolids Rule.[85] However, these regulations are not iron-clad, and in some cases, biosolids may be land applied against US EPA guidelines before heavy metal test results are available,[86] and some metals/metalloids such as boron and silver, for which the health implications are not well understood, remain unregulated.[60]

Pesticides

Prevalence of pesticides

Pesticides are widely used in US agriculture to increase crop yield and meet food demands. In 2012, more than 1 billion pounds of pesticides were applied in agricultural fields, with herbicides accounting for the largest share (63%), followed by fumigants (12%), fungicides (6%), and insecticides (4%) (**Box 4**).[87]

Routes of childhood exposure to pesticides

Widespread use of pesticides results in ubiquitous exposure among US children, largely from consumption of pesticide-contaminated food.[88] However, children living in agricultural communities, where 90% of pesticides are currently used in the United States,[89] are at particular risk. Children living on or near farmland are exposed to pesticides via drift from treated fields to nearby homes or schools[90]; take-home exposures (in which workers who have handled or been in contact with pesticides inadvertently carry substances into homes and vehicles on clothing or footwear)[91]; or consumption of contaminated water.[92] Children living near areas sprayed with pesticides can also be exposed via direct contamination of their possessions, food, or water.[93]

Health effects of pesticide exposure

Acute pesticide poisonings are relatively uncommon in US children,[94] but exposure to pesticides has been linked to a broad range of chronic pediatric adverse health

Box 4
Common pesticides applied in agricultural fields by category

Herbicides
- Glyphosate (eg, Roundup)
- Atrazine
- 2,4-dichlorophenoxyacetic acid

Insecticides
- Neonicotinoids
- Pyrethroids
- Organophosphate pesticides (eg, chlorpyrifos)

Fungicides
- Mancozeb
- Chlorothalonil

Fumigants
- Dichloropropene
- Metam
- Metam potassium
- Methyl bromide

effects. Organophosphate (OP) pesticides, carbamates, and pyrethroids have been associated with cognitive and behavioral problems, including attention-deficit/hyperactivity and autism spectrum disorders.[89,95–98] Exposure to OP pesticides and pyrethroids in early life has been associated with poorer lung function and respiratory symptomatology in school-age children.[99,100] Home insecticide and herbicide use has been linked to childhood cancers such as leukemia,[101] neuroblastoma,[102] and brain cancer.[103] Emerging literature suggests that exposure to current use pesticides, such as glyphosate, may be associated with obesity and cardiometabolic outcomes, and IARC designates these as "probably carcinogenic to humans."[104,105]

GUIDANCE FOR CLINICIANS

The AAP recommends taking an environmental history, including questions about diet, household, and occupational exposures, as a key component of pediatric preventive health care.[106] Accordingly, the Western States Pediatric Environmental Health Specialty Unit (PEHSU) has developed an online tool with environmental health anticipatory guidance by child age[107] to supplement the AAP's Bright Futures Guidelines.[108]

We recommend that pediatric clinicians practicing in rural areas ask families specifically about home wood stove use, water sources, and agricultural exposures. These questions could be integrated into clinic workflow by the clinician during the visit, a member of the clinical team during rooming, or reported by patients on written materials. For patients who screen positive, we recommend that clinicians provide families with specific anticipatory guidance during the visit and detailed resources (**Table 1**), as studies indicate that clinician guidance is key in helping families mitigate environmental exposures.[27]

Pediatric clinicians can also help families navigate subsequent testing for contaminants and appropriate medical monitoring and management. Blood testing for various contaminants may be available through state or private laboratories, and often state Departments of Health are able to provide testing-related information. An invaluable resource is the national PEHSU, a network of experts in health conditions associated with environmental exposures who are available to consult with clinicians and families.[109] Further information on toxicologic profiles and health effects is available through the ATSDR, which offers continuing education for clinicians.[110] While many of the contaminants described in this review may be unfamiliar to generalist pediatric clinicians, often the subsequent medical monitoring after an environmental exposure is well within the realm of primary care.

Finally, clinicians can also be invaluable "scholar activists," lending their frontline experiences and clinical expertise to nonprofit and governmental bodies seeking to advance environmental justice.[10,13]

EXACERBATING FACTORS AND OTHER CONSIDERATIONS

Children living in rural communities are often simultaneously exposed to environmental pollutants from wood stove use, well water, and farming practices, as evidenced by the high prevalence of 2 or more of these in a specific state (see **Fig. 2**). Future studies need to consider joint environmental exposures in rural communities, as the impact of one exposure in the presence of another may be amplified beyond their independent effects on health outcomes.[111] Given their low population density and distance from large population centers, rural areas are often the target of undesirable land uses, such as hazardous industries and waste,[112] which may escalate the amount and degree of contaminants in well water and biosolids.

Table 1
Specific anticipatory guidance and resources for children who may have rural environmental exposures

Exposure	Anticipatory Guidance	Resources
Wood Stove	• Burn only dry wood • Remove ashes regularly • Maintain annual chimney cleaning and inspection	• Best practices for burning wood: https://www.epa.gov/burnwise • Find installation and maintenance professionals: https://www.csia.org/or https://www.nficertified.org/
	• Install an air filter	• Guide to air cleaners in the home: https://www.epa.gov/indoor-air-quality-iaq/guide-air-cleaners-home
	• Replace old stoves with newer, the Environmental Protection Agency(EPA)-certified wood stoves	• EPA certified wood and pellet stoves: https://www.epa.gov/compliance/epa-certified-wood-heater-database
Well Water	• Baseline tests[1]: ○ Coliform bacteria ○ Nitrates ○ Lead ○ Fluoride ○ Arsenic ○ Radon ○ Other (location-specific, consult local department of health) • Annual tests: ○ Coliform bacteria ○ Nitrates	• EPA guidance on testing private wells: https://www.epa.gov/privatewells/protect-your-homes-water#welltestanchor • Centers for Disease Control and Prevention (CDC) guidance on testing private wells: https://www.cdc.gov/healthywater/drinking/private/wells/testing.html
	• If tests show levels are high, you can: ○ Identify any structural defects ○ Remediation may be possible via treatment or filtration	• EPA emergency disinfection of drinking water: https://www.epa.gov/ground-water-and-drinking-water/emergency-disinfection-drinking-water • CDC guide to drinking water treatment: https://www.cdc.gov/healthywater/drinking/home-water-treatment/household_water_treatment.html

Farm-Biosolids (Sludge) Farm-Biosolids (Sludge) Continued	Determining exposure: • Check with state environmental agencies about location of sludge spreading sites Known or suspected exposure: • Test water source(s) for perfluoroalkyl and polyfluoroalkyl substances (PFAS) • Check with local and state agencies for water testing and reimbursement • Consider testing serum PFAS levels Reduce exposure if source is known: • Consider alternate sources of water • Install an National Sanitation Foundation (NSF)-certified water filter • Follow local wild game, fish, and farmed food consumption advisories	• EPA basic information about biosolids: https://www.epa.gov/biosolids • Find state contacts and EPA certified laboratories for testing drinking water: https://www.epa.gov/dwlabcert/contact-information-certification-programs-and-certified-laboratories-drinking-water • Clinical guidance for PFAS exposure, testing, and medical monitoring: https://nap.nationalacademies.org/catalog/26156/guidance-on-pfas-exposure-testing-and-clinical-follow-up • PFAS information for clinicians: https://www.atsdr.cdc.gov/pfas/resources/pfas-information-for-clinicians.html • Filter and water treatment information: https://www.cdc.gov/healthywater/drinking/home-water-treatment/water-filters.html • Find NSF certified water filters: https://info.nsf.org/Certified/dwtu/
Farm- Pesticides	• Living near a farm that uses pesticides: ○ Close windows and keep children indoors when pesticides are being sprayed on nearby fields • Living with a person who works on a farm that uses pesticides: ○ Wash hands and face and change out of contaminated clothes and shoes before returning home or entering a car ○ Wash work clothes separately from the rest of the laundry • Consuming water and food contaminated with pesticides: ○ Eat organic when possible, but not at the expense of a healthy diet rich in fruits and vegetables ○ Use the Environmental Working Group (EWG) Food Guide to determine produce with the highest and lowest levels of pesticide residue ○ Wash and scrub produce with water, throw away outer leaves of leafy vegetables, and trim skin and fat from fish and meats where pesticides can accumulate	• Pediatric environmental toolkit: pesticides: https://peht.ucsf.edu/search.php?pane=reference&topic=pesticides • EPA agricultural workers pesticide safety: https://www.epa.gov/pesticide-worker-safety • EWG Shoppers Guide: http://www.ewg.org/foodnews

Environmental hazards in rural life may exacerbate health disparities between children living in rural and urban areas. Rural children have less access to health care, fewer primary care physicians per capita, and a greater uninsured population than children living in urban areas[113,114]; hence, they are less likely to receive preventive health care. Children living in rural areas also face a unique set of psychosocial stressors including discrimination and stigma; geographic and social isolation; and housing and food insecurity,[115,116] which may increase susceptibility to the effects of environmental exposures and lead to synergistic impacts on health outcomes,[111] such as neurodevelopmental and mental disorders.

Importantly, effects of climate change such as flooding, drought, wildfires, and extreme heat may act synergistically with existing rural environmental hazards to exacerbate health effects. For example, extreme rainfall and increasing water temperatures may facilitate well water contamination,[117] while drought conditions can concentrate contaminants in well water.[118] In addition, climate-related events can affect crop uptake, environmental distribution, and toxicities of pesticides and other chemical contaminants.[117,119] Moreover, climate-related migration is likely to drive more of the US population toward rural and less climate-sensitive areas,[120] underscoring the need for increased awareness of rural environmental exposures.

Future work should also focus on approaches to better mitigate these exposures, more quickly reduce body burdens following exposure, and support mental and physical resilience in affected communities. Finally, as more pediatric clinicians communicate guidance on these rural exposures to their patients and their guardians, it is key to assess and improve environmental health literacy among these populations.

SUMMARY

Environmental exposures to wood stove smoke, contaminated well water, and agricultural pollutants pose unique health risks to children living in rural communities. Contaminants from these exposures encompass a range of pollutants that can have short-term and long-term health effects including poor respiratory health, obesity and cardiometabolic dysfunction, neurodevelopmental disorders, and cancer. Children are more susceptible to these exposures, and their unique physiology places them at higher risk of long-term health consequences as compared to adults. Pediatric clinicians can play a key role in screening children for risk of environmental exposures and providing families with essential resources on exposure mitigation and medical monitoring.

CLINICS CARE POINTS

- Pediatric clinicians should incorporate environmental health screening for children living in rural areas that includes screening for exposure to smoke from wood stoves, contaminated well water, and agricultural pollutants.
- Patients who screen positive for these environmental health exposures may be at increased risk for certain health conditions.
- For patients who screen positive, pediatric clinicians should offer exposure reduction advice as outlined in this review and work with local and national resources such as Departments of Health, Pediatric Environmental Health Specialty Units, and the Agency for Toxic Substances and Disease Registry.

DISCLOSURES

The authors have received support from the National Institutes of Health, United States (R01ES030101, R21ES035596, T42 OH008416, NCI 5T32CA134286-13). The authors have nothing to disclose.

REFERENCES

1. Davis JC, Rupasingha A, Cromartie J, et al. Rural America at a glance. 2022 Edition. US Department of Agriculture Economic Research Service; 2022.
2. Jones CC. Environmental justice in rural context: Land-application of biosolids in central Virginia. Environ Justice 2011;4(1).
3. Pellow DN. Environmental justice and rural studies: A critical conversation and invitation to collaboration. J Rural Stud 2016;47:381–6.
4. Theis N, Driscoll A. Rural consciousness and framing environmental (in)justice. Environ Justice 2023;16(2):118–25.
5. Miller MD, Marty MA, Arcus A, et al. Differences Between Children and Adults: Implications for Risk Assessment at California EPA. Int J Toxicol 2002;21(5): 403–18.
6. Rokoff LB, Koutrakis P, Garshick E, et al. Wood Stove Pollution in the Developed World: A Case to Raise Awareness Among Pediatricians. Curr Probl Pediatr Adolesc Health Care 2017;47(6):123–41.
7. Bateson TF, Schwartz J. Children's response to air pollutants. J Toxicol Environ Health 2007;71(3):238–43.
8. Johnson-Restrepo B, Kannan K. An assessment of sources and pathways of human exposure to polybrominated diphenyl ethers in the United States. Chemosphere 2009;76(4):542–8.
9. Carroquino MJ, Posada M, Landrigan P. Environmental Toxicology: Children at Risk. Environ Toxicol 2012;239–91. Published online December 4.
10. Budolfson KC, Etzel RA. Climate change and child health equity. Pediatr Clin N Am 2023;70:837–53.
11. Criswell R, Wang Y, Christensen B, et al. Concentrations of per- and polyfluoroalkyl substances in paired maternal plasma and human milk in the New Hampshire Birth Cohort. Env Sci Technol 2023;57(1):463–72.
12. Heindel JJ, Newbold R, Schug TT. Endocrine disruptors and obesity. Nat Rev Endocrinol 2015;11(11):653–61.
13. Trasande L, Kassotis CD. The pediatrician's role in protecting children from environmnetal hazards. Pediatr Clin N Am 2023;70:137–50.
14. U.S. Energy Information Administration - EIA - Independent Statistics and Analysis. Form EIA-457A 2020 RECS Survey Data. Available at: https://www.eia.gov/consumption/residential/data/2020/#fueluses. [Accessed 25 October 2023].
15. US Census Bureau. Table H2: Urban and Rural. 2022. Available at: https://data.census.gov/table/DECENNIALDHC2020.H2?q=urban+race&y=2020&d=DEC+Demographic+and+Housing+Characteristics&tp=true. [Accessed 25 October 2023].
16. USFS Tree Canopy Cover Datasets. Available at: https://data.fs.usda.gov/geodata/rastergateway/treecanopycover/.
17. US Census Bureau. House Heating Fuel - Table B25040. 2022. Available at: https://data.census.gov/table/ACSDT1Y2022.B25040?q=fuel&g=010XX00US$0400000&moe=false&tp=true. [Accessed 25 October 2023].
18. Naeher LP, Brauer M, Lipsett M, et al. Woodsmoke health effects: a review. Inhal Toxicol 2007;19(1):67–106.

19. Balmes JR. When smoke gets in your lungs. Proc Am Thorac Soc. 7(2):98-101.
20. Fleisch AF, Rokoff LB, Garshick E, et al. Residential Wood Stove Use and Indoor Exposure to PM2.5 and its Components in Northern New England. J Expo Sci Environ Epidemiol 2020;30(2):350–61.
21. Grahame TJ, Klemm R, Schlesinger RB. Public health and components of particulate matter: the changing assessment of black carbon. J Air Waste Manag Assoc 1995 2014;64(6):620–60.
22. Noonan CW, Ward TJ, Semmens EO. Estimating the Number of Vulnerable People in the United States Exposed to Residential Wood Smoke. Environ Health Perspect 2015;123(2):A30.
23. Garcia E, Rice MB, Gold DR. Air pollution and lung function in children. J Allergy Clin Immunol 2021;148(1):1–14.
24. Mehta SS, Elizabeth Hodgson M, Lunn RM, et al. Indoor wood-burning from stoves and fireplaces and incident lung cancer among Sister Study participants. Environ Int 2023;178:108128.
25. International Agency for Research on Cancer. Iarc - household use of solid fuels and high-temperature frying 2010. Published online.
26. Fleisch AF, Seshasayee SM, Garshick E, et al. Assessment of Maternal Glycemia and Newborn Size Among Pregnant Women Who Use Wood Stoves in Northern New England. JAMA Netw Open 2020;3(5):e206046.
27. Murray A, Hall A, Weaver J, et al. Methods for estimating locations of housing units served by private domestic wells in the United States applied to 2010. JAWRA J Am Water Resour Assoc 2021;57(5):828–43.
28. Johnson T, Belitz K. Domestic well locations and populations served in the contiguous U.S.: 1990. Sci Total Environ 2017;607-608:658–68.
29. Census US. Historical Census of Housing Tables: Source of Water. Census.gov. Available at: https://www.census.gov/data/tables/time-series/dec/coh-water.html. [Accessed 2 February 2024].
30. O'Neill HS, Flanagan SV, Gleason JA, et al. Targeted private well outreach following a change in drinking water standard: Arsenic and the New Jersey Private Well Testing Act. J Public Health Manag Pract JPHMP 2023;29(1):E29–36.
31. Woolf AD, Stierman BD, Barnett ED, et al, Council on environmental health and climate change, committee on infectious diseases, COMMITTEE ON INFECTIOUS DISEASES. Drinking water from private wells and risks to children. Pediatrics 2023;151(2). https://doi.org/10.1542/peds.2022-060644. e2022060644.
32. NH Department of Health and Human Services. *NH Private Well Water Summary, 2015.* NH Environmental Public Health Tracking Program. Bureau of Public Health Statistics & Informatics, Division of Public Health Services 2015.
33. MacDonald K, Tippett M. Reducing public exposure to common, harmful well water contaminants through targeted outreach to highly susceptible neighborhoods as a method of increasing the likelihood of testing and treatment of water from private wells. J Water Health 2020;18(4):522–32.
34. Malecki KMC, Schultz AA, Severtson DJ, et al. Private-well stewardship among a general population based sample of private well-owners. Sci Total Environ 2017;601-602:1533–43.
35. Elliott EG, Ettinger AS, Leaderer BP, et al. A systematic evaluation of chemicals in hydraulic-fracturing fluids and wastewater for reproductive and developmental toxicity. J Expo Sci Environ Epidemiol 2017;27:90–9.
36. Richardson SD. Disinfection by-products and other emerging contaminants in drinking water. Trends Anal Chem 2003;22(10):666–84.

37. Division of Environmental Health. Drinking water PFAS concentrations and exposure factors influencing measured and predicted serum PFAS concentrations. Michigan Department of Health and Human Services; 2024.
38. IARC. IARC - A Review of Human Carcinogens. Vol 100F.; 2012.
39. IARC. IARC - Ingested Nitrate and Nitrite, and Cyanobacterial Peptide Toxins. Vol 94.; 2010.
40. IARC. IARC - Inorganic and Organic Lead Compounds. Vol 87.; 2006.
41. IARC. IARC - Selenium and Selenium Compounds. Vol 135.; 1987.
42. ATSDR. Toxicological profile for uranium. U.S. Department of Health and Human Services, Public Health Service; 2013.
43. ATDSR. Toxicological profile for arsenic. U.S. Department of Health and Human Services, Public Health Service; 2007.
44. US EPA. Arsenic, inorganic. National Center for Environmental Assessment; 2023. Available at: https://cfpub.epa.gov/ncea/iris_drafts/recordisplay.cfm?deid=253756#tab-3. [Accessed 30 January 2024].
45. Bellinger D, Sloman J, Leviton A, et al. Low-level lead exposure and children's cognitive function in the preschool years. Pediatrics 1991;87(2):219–27.
46. Canfield RL, Henderson Jr CR, Cory-Slechta DA, et al. Intellectual impairment in children with blood lead concentrations below 10 microg per deciliter. N Engl J Med 2003;348(16):1517–26.
47. Chen A, Cai B, Dietrich KN, et al. Lead exposure, IQ, and behavior in urban 5-7 year olds: Does lead affect behavior only by lowering IQ? Pediatrics 2007; 119(3):e650–8.
48. Tellez-Rojo M, Bellinger D, Arroyo-Quiroz C, et al. Longitudinal associations between blood lead concentrations lower than 10 microg/dL and neurobehavioral development in environmentally exposed children in Mexico City. Pediatrics 2006;118(2):e323–30.
49. Laclaustra M, Navas-Acien A, Stranges S, et al. Serum selenium concentrations and hypertension in the US population. Circ Cardiovasc Qual Outcomes 2009;2: 369–76.
50. Keen C, Zidenberg-Cherr S. Manganese. In: *Encyclopedia of food Sciences and nutrition*. Second. Academic Press; 2003. p. 3686–91.
51. Henn BC, Schnaas L, Ettinger AS, et al. Associations of Early Childhood Manganese and Lead Coexposure with Neurodevelopment. Environ Health Perspect 2011;120(1):126–31.
52. Bouchard MF, Sauve S, Barbeau B, et al. Intellectual Impairment in School-Age Children Exposed to Manganese from Drinking Water. Environ Health Perspect 2011;119(1):138–43.
53. Henn BC, Ettinger AS, Schwartz J, et al. Early Postnatal Blood Manganese Levels and Children's Neurodevelopment. Epidemiology 2011;21(4):433–9.
54. Menezes-Filho JA, de O Novaes C, Moreira JC, et al. Elevated manganese and cognitive performance in school-aged children and their mothers. Environ Res 2011;111(1):156–63.
55. Riojas-Rodriguez H, Solis-Vivanco R, Schilmann A, et al. Intellectual function in Mexican children living in a mining area and environmentally exposed to manganese. Environ Health Perspect 2010;118(10):1465–70.
56. USDA. Farm and land in farms, 2021 summary. United States Department of Agriculture, Natural Agricultural Statistics Service; 2022. Available at: https://www.nass.usda.gov/Publications/Todays_Reports/reports/fnlo0222.pdf. [Accessed 2 February 2024].

57. US Forest Service. USDA, Inventoried Roadless Area Acreage by State. Available at: https://www.fs.usda.gov/Internet/FSE_DOCUMENTS/fsm8_037652.htm. [Accessed 2 February 2024].
58. Cybersecurity and Infrastructure Security Agency. Water and Wastewater Systems. US Department of Homeland Security. Available at: https://www.cisa.gov/topics/critical-infrastructure-security-and-resilience/critical-infrastructure-sectors/water-and-wastewater-sector#:~:text=There%20are%20approximately%20153%2C000%20public,systems%20in%20the%20United%20States. Accessed January 30, 2024.
59. US EPA O. Biosolids Generation, Use, and Disposal in the United States. 2018. Available at: https://www.epa.gov/biosolids/biosolids-generation-use-and-disposal-united-states. [Accessed 20 October 2023].
60. A National Biosolids Regulation. Quality, End Use & Disposal Survey: Final Report. 2007. Available at: http://static1.squarespace.com/static/54806478e4b0dc44e1698e88/t/5488541fe4b03c0a9b8ee09b/1418220575693/NtlBiosolidsReport-20July07.pdf.
61. Seiple TE, Coleman AM, Skaggs RL. Municipal wastewater sludge as a sustainable bioresource in the United States. J Environ Manage 2017;197:673–80.
62. Mills M. Session 6: PFAS Treatment in Biosolids – State of the Science.
63. National Academies of Sciences, Engineering, and Medicine. Guidance on PFAS exposure, testing, and clinical follow-up. The National Academies Press; 2022.
64. Maine Department of Environmental Protection. PFAS and Maine DEP. 2023. Available at: https://www.maine.gov/dep/spills/topics/pfas/maine-pfas.html.
65. Maine Department of Inland Fisheries and Wildlife. PFAS Do Not Eat Advisory: For Deer and Wild Turkey in Portions of Fairfield and Skowhegan. 2023. Available at: https://www.maine.gov/ifw/hunting-trapping/hunting/laws-rules/pfas-related-consumption-advisory.html. [Accessed 14 December 2023].
66. Pozzebon EA, Seifert L. Emerging environmental health risks associated with the land application of biosolids: a scoping review. Environ Health 2023;22:57.
67. Naderi Beni N, Karimifard S, Gilley J, et al. Higher concentrations of microplastics in runoff from biosolid-amended croplands than manure-amended croplands. Commun Earth Environ 2023;4(1):1–9.
68. Armitage J, Cousins IT, Buck RC, et al. Modeling Global-Scale Fate and Transport of Perfluorooctanoate Emitted from Direct Sources. Environ Sci Technol 2006;40(22):6969–75.
69. Olsen GW, Burris JM, Ehresman DJ, et al. Half-life of serum elimination of perfluorooctanesulfonate,perfluorohexanesulfonate, and perfluorooctanoate in retired fluorochemical production workers. Environ Health Perspect 2007;115(9):1298–305.
70. Agency for Toxic Substances and Disease Registry. PFAS Information for Clinicians - 2024. 2024. Available at: https://www.atsdr.cdc.gov/pfas/resources/pfas-information-for-clinicians.html. [Accessed 16 February 2024].
71. Toxicological profile for perfluoroalkyls. doi:10.15620/cdc:59198.
72. Zahm S, Bonde JP, Chiu WA, et al. Carcinogenicity of perfluorooctanoic acid (PFOA) and perfluorooctanesulfonic acid (PFOS). Lancet Oncol 2024;25(1):16–7.
73. Vethaak AD, Legler J. Microplastics and human health. Science 2021;371(6530):672–4.
74. Wang YL, Lee YH, Hsu YH, et al. The Kidney-Related Effects of Polystyrene Microplastics on Human Kidney Proximal Tubular Epithelial Cells HK-2 and Male C57BL/6 Mice. Environ Health Perspect 2021;129(5):057003.

75. Leusch FDL, Ziajahromi S. Converting mg/L to Particles/L: Reconciling the Occurrence and Toxicity Literature on Microplastics. Environ Sci Technol 2021;55(17):11470–2.
76. Ji J, Wu X, Li X, et al. Effects of microplastics in aquatic environments on inflammatory bowel disease. Environ Res 2023;229:115974.
77. Yan Z, Liu Y, Zhang T, et al. Analysis of Microplastics in Human Feces Reveals a Correlation between Fecal Microplastics and Inflammatory Bowel Disease Status. Environ Sci Technol 2022;56(1):414–21.
78. Qian N, Gao X, Lang X, et al. Rapid single-plastic chemical imaging of nanoplastics by SRS microscopy. Proc Natl Acad Sci USA 2024;121(3). e2300582121.
79. Black GP, Anumol T, Young TM. Analyzing a broader spectrum of endocrine active organic contaminants in sewage sludge with High Resolution LC-QTOF-MS suspect screening and QSAR toxicity prediction. Environ Sci Process Impacts 2019;21(7):1099–114.
80. De Coster S, van Larebeke N. Endocrine-Disrupting Chemicals: Associated Disorders and Mechanisms of Action. J Environ Public Health 2012;2012:713696.
81. Ondon BS, Li S, Zhou Q, et al. Sources of Antibiotic Resistant Bacteria (ARB) and Antibiotic Resistance Genes (ARGs) in the Soil: A Review of the Spreading Mechanism and Human Health Risks. Rev Environ Contam Toxicol 2021;256: 121–53.
82. Endocrine active substances | EFSA. 2023. Available at: https://www.efsa.europa.eu/en/topics/topic/endocrine-active-substances. [Accessed 18 October 2023].
83. Venkatesan AK, Halden RU. National Inventory of Alkylphenol Ethoxylate Compounds in U.S. Sewage Sludges and Chemical Fate in Outdoor Soil Mesocosms. Environ Pollut Barking Essex 1987 2013;174:189–93.
84. Acir IH, Guenther K. Endocrine-disrupting metabolites of alkylphenol ethoxylates – A critical review of analytical methods, environmental occurrences, toxicity, and regulation. Sci Total Environ 2018;635:1530–46.
85. A Plain English Guide to the EPA Part 503 Biosolids Rule.
86. Iranpour: Regulations for biosolids land application. - Google Scholar. Available at: https://scholar.google.com/scholar_lookup?title=Regulations%20for%20biosolids%20land%20application%20in%20US%20and%20European%20Union&publication_year=2004&author=R.%20Iranpour&author=H.H.J.%20Cox&author=R.J.%20Kearney&author=J.H.%20Clark&author=A.B.%20Pincince&author=G.T.%20Daigger. [Accessed 11 October 2023].
87. Atwood D, Paisley-Jones C. Pesticides industry sales and usage: 2008–2012 market estimates. US Environmental Protection Agency; 2017. Available at: https://www.epa.gov/sites/default/files/2017-01/documents/pesticides-industry-sales-usage-2016_0.pdf. [Accessed 13 October 2023].
88. Council on Environmental Health, Roberts JR, Karr CJ, et al. Pesticide Exposure in Children. Pediatrics 2012;130(6):e1757–63.
89. Schafer K, Marquez E. A generation in jeopardy: how pesticides are undermining our children's health and intelligence. Pesticide Action Network North America; 2012. Available at: https://www.panna.org/wp-content/uploads/2022/12/KidsHealthReportOct2012.pdf. [Accessed 13 October 2023].
90. Deziel NC, Friesen MC, Hoppin JA, et al. A Review of Nonoccupational Pathways for Pesticide Exposure in Women Living in Agricultural Areas. Environ Health Perspect 2015;123(6):515–24.

91. López-Gálvez W, Quirós-Alcalá, Quirós-Alcalá L, et al. Systematic Literature Review of the Take-Home Route of Pesticide Exposure via Biomonitoring and Environmental Monitoring. Int J Environ Res Publ Health 2019;16(12):2177.
92. USGS Fact. Sheet 1995–244: pesticide in ground water. U.S. Geological Survey; 1996. Available at: https://pubs.usgs.gov/fs/1995/0244/. [Accessed 27 October 2023].
93. Eskenazi B, Levine DI, Rauch S, et al. A community-based education programme to reduce insecticide exposure from indoor residual spraying in Limpopo, South Africa. Malar J 2019;18(1):199.
94. Gummin DD, Mowry JB, Beuhler MC, et al. 2021 Annual Report of the National Poison Data System © (NPDS) from America's Poison Centers: 39th Annual Report. Clin Toxicol 2022;60(12):1381–643.
95. Dórea JG. Exposure to environmental neurotoxic substances and neurodevelopment in children from Latin America and the Caribbean. Environ Res 2021; 192:110199.
96. Hertz-Picciotto I, Sass JB, Engel S, et al. Organophosphate exposures during pregnancy and child neurodevelopment: Recommendations for essential policy reforms. PLoS Med 2018;15(10):e1002671.
97. Vrijheid M, Casas M, Gascon M, et al. Environmental pollutants and child health—A review of recent concerns. Int J Hyg Environ Health 2016;219(4–5): 331–42.
98. Andersen HR, David A, Freire C, et al. Pyrethroids and developmental neurotoxicity - A critical review of epidemiological studies and supporting mechanistic evidence. Environ Res 2022;214:113935.
99. Buralli RJ, Dultra AF, Ribeiro H. Respiratory and Allergic Effects in Children Exposed to Pesticides—A Systematic Review. Int J Environ Res Publ Health 2020;17(8):2740.
100. Gilden RC, Harris RL, Friedmann EJ, et al. Systematic Review: Association of Pesticide Exposure and Child Wheeze and Asthma. Curr Pediatr Rev 2023; 19(2):169–78.
101. Karalexi MA, Tagkas CF, Markozannes G, et al. Exposure to pesticides and childhood leukemia risk: A systematic review and meta-analysis. Environ Pollut 2021;285:117376.
102. Hymel E, Degarege A, Fritch J, et al. Agricultural exposures and risk of childhood neuroblastoma: a systematic review and meta-analysis. Environ Sci Pollut Res 2023. https://doi.org/10.1007/s11356-023-30315-z.
103. Feulefack J, Khan A, Forastiere F, et al. Parental Pesticide Exposure and Childhood Brain Cancer: A Systematic Review and Meta-Analysis Confirming the IARC/WHO Monographs on Some Organophosphate Insecticides and Herbicides. Children 2021;8(12):1096.
104. Guyton K, Loomis D, Yann G, et al. Carcinogenicity of tetrachlorvinphos, parathion, malathion, diazinon, and glycophosphate. Lancet Oncol 2015;16(5):490–1.
105. Eskenazi B, Gunier RB, Rauch S, et al. Association of Lifetime Exposure to Glyphosate and Aminomethylphosphonic Acid (AMPA) with Liver Inflammation and Metabolic Syndrome at Young Adulthood: Findings from the CHAMACOS Study. Environ Health Perspect 2023;131(3):037001.
106. Taking an Environmental History. Available at: https://www.aap.org/en/patient-care/environmental-health/promoting-healthy-environments-for-children/taking-an-environmental-history/. [Accessed 18 October 2023].
107. Pediatric Environmental Health Toolkit. Available at: https://peht.ucsf.edu/home.php. [Accessed 18 October 2023].

108. Bright Futures. Available at: https://www.aap.org/en/practice-management/bright-futures/. [Accessed 18 October 2023].
109. Pediatric Environmental Health Specialty Units. 2023. Available at: https://www.pehsu.net. [Accessed 14 December 2023].
110. Agency for Toxic Substances and Disease Registry. 2023. Available at: https://www.atsdr.cdc.gov. [Accessed 14 December 2023].
111. Rider CV, Simmons JE, Birnbaum LS. Chemical Mixtures and Combined Chemical and Nonchemical Stressors: Exposure, . Toxicity, analysis, and risk. Springer International Publishing; 2018.
112. Johnston J, Cushing L. Chemical Exposures, Health, and Environmental Justice in Communities Living on the Fenceline of Industry. Curr Environ Health Rep 2020;7(1):48–57.
113. Coughlin SS, Clary C, Johnson JA, et al. Continuing challenges in rural health in the United States. J Env Health Sci 2019;5(2):90–2.
114. Gong G, Phillips SG, Hudson C, et al. Higher US rural mortality rates linked to socioeconomic status, physician shortages, and lack of health insurance. Health Aff (Millwood) 2019;38(12).
115. Coleman-Jensen A, Steffen B. Food Insecurity and Housing Insecurity. In: Rural poverty in the United States. Columbia University Press; 2017.
116. Morales DA, Barksdale CL, Beckel-Mitchener AC. A call to action to address rural mental health disparities. J Clin Transl Sci 2020;4(5):463–7.
117. Noyes PD, McElwee MK, Miller HD, et al. The toxicology of climate change: Environmental contaminants in a warming world. Environ Int 2009;35(6):971–86.
118. American Academy of Pediatrics C on EH and C of ID, Committee on Infectious Diseases, Rogan WJ, et al. Drinking water from private wells and risks to children. Pediatrics 2009;123(6):1599–605.
119. Muehe EM, Wang T, Kerl CF, et al. Rice production threatened by coupled stresses of climate and soil arsenic. Nat Commun 2019;10:4985.
120. Fan X, Miao C, Duan Q, et al. Future Climate Change Hotspots Under Different 21st Century Warming Scenarios. Earth's Future 2021;9(6). e2021EF002027.

Social Vulnerability of Pediatric Populations Living in Ambulance Deserts

Yvonne Jonk, PhD[a,b,*], Heidi O'Connor, MS[b,c], Tyler DeAngelis, BA[b], Celia Jewell, RN, MPH[b,c], Erika Ziller, PhD[d]

KEYWORDS

• Ambulance deserts • Rural health • Socioeconomic • Poverty • Uninsurance • Mortality risk

KEY POINTS

- An ambulance desert (AD) is defined as a populated area outside of a 25-minute drive time from where an ambulance is located.
- Many (approximately 20%) of those in rural areas living in ambulance deserts are children.
- Children living in ADs are also challenged by having a greater proportion of adverse social determinants of health, such as poverty and uninsurance.
- The potential for adverse health outcomes among vulnerable children experiencing acute illness or injury within ADs deserves further study.

INTRODUCTION

Of the 4.5 million people living in areas of the United States with limited access to ambulance services (referred to as ambulance deserts [ADs]), approximately 1 in 5 (20%) are children aged 18 years and younger.[1] Ambulance deserts are defined as populated areas in the United States that are not accessible within 25 minutes of where an ambulance is stationed.[2] This lack of timely response to a 911 call by emergency medical service (EMS) providers can result in serious adverse health consequences, including death, for children and families facing an acute illness or injury.

Most people expect that when they call 911 an ambulance staffed by trained professionals will come to their aid within a reasonable time frame, and then treat and

[a] Department of Public Health, Muskie School of Public Service, University of Southern Maine, 222 Wishcamper Center, 34 Bedford Street, PO Box 9300, Portland, ME 04104, USA; [b] Maine Rural Health Research Center, University of Southern Maine, Portland, ME, USA; [c] Department of Public Health, Muskie School of Public Service, University of Southern Maine, Portland, ME, USA; [d] Health Services Research Center, Larner College of Medicine, University of Vermont, Burlington, VT, USA

* Corresponding author.
E-mail address: yvonne.jonk@maine.edu

Pediatr Clin N Am 72 (2025) 85–92
https://doi.org/10.1016/j.pcl.2024.07.039 pediatric.theclinics.com

transport them to the nearest hospital or emergency department if necessary. Unfortunately, this expectation is limited to communities that have the resources necessary to support an ambulance service and that have community members who are willing and able to staff their local ambulance service, often on a volunteer basis.[3–5] Less than 10% of ambulance services are affiliated with local hospitals or clinics[6–8] and have not been well integrated into the health care sector(s). The reasons for this lack of integration are in part linked to how ambulance services were originally regulated and funded. The gaps in coverage illustrated by the AD study have provided evidence that the current regulations governing ambulance service provision are not adequately supporting and reimbursing ambulance services and are in need of reform.

Historically, ambulance services have been viewed as a transportation service and overseen by the US Department of Transportation.[9] With the technological development of portable medical devices and procedures, ambulance services have transitioned from a transportation role to the provision of medical services, capable of saving lives and administering care out in the field. Unfortunately, much of the care provided by EMS providers is not billed and paid for by health insurance carriers. Insurance reimbursement for prehospital services has been limited to instances when EMS providers bring patients to the hospital or emergency department.[10] However, EMS providers not only play a critical role in caring for patients experiencing a traumatic injury or illness, but they also serve an important role in responding to calls and caring for patients who do not need to be hospitalized or brought to the emergency department.

In addition to the fact that the EMS field has been evolving and is gaining recognition as an important component of the health care infrastructure, rural areas face additional challenges when it comes to financial sustainability. Even if insurance carriers and third-party payors were to reimburse EMS providers for responding to all 911 calls and for providing health care and/or public health services out in the community, other issues make it challenging for ambulance services to sustain themselves financially. The low volume problem that has plagued rural hospitals and clinics is also an issue for EMS providers. EMS providers are not typically reimbursed for time spent on call and time spent behind the wheel when responding to calls. Driving long distances round trip in remote rural areas, along with supporting the high fixed costs associated with equipping ambulances with the latest technology has made it difficult for ambulance services to break even.[11] The high fixed and variable costs associated with setting up a rural ambulance service, and training/maintaining EMS certification, has led to many communities imposing mill levies, collecting donations, and holding fundraising activities to support their local ambulance service(s).

Many communities have been relying on volunteers willing to take on the costs associated with training and certification. Aging rural communities, along with the out-migration of young people, has led to the erosion of rural communities' volunteer base,[12,13] leading to many ambulance services closing because of staffing shortages.

The combination of these factors has led to gaps in the provision of ambulance services known as ADs. Prior work funded by the Federal Office of Rural Health Policy (FORHP) within the Health Resources and Services Administration (HRSA) has documented that ADs are more likely to exist in rural areas. Because Maine ranks among the most rural states in the nation, researchers at the Maine Rural Health Research Center have a strong interest in determining the extent to which rural pediatric populations live in ADs and identify the socioeconomic risk factors associated with living in ADs nationwide.

The next section discusses the unique needs of rural pediatric populations, and the risks associated with lacking adequate EMS services trained to care for pediatric patients. This is followed by the authors' findings from a state-level analysis of the variation in the socioeconomic characteristics of pediatric populations living in ADs. Finally, the need for reform options that will facilitate expanding the footprint of EMS providers in rural communities is discussed.

DISCUSSION

Rural Pediatric Health and Health-Related Social Needs

Previous studies have documented that rural children are more likely to live in poverty,[14] live in primary care and mental health professional shortage areas,[15] and have limited access to dental[16] and telehealth services,[17] as well as suicide prevention or family crisis services.[18]

Pediatric Mortality Risks

A recent study (2021) found that rural children tend to be at higher risk of death due to unintentional injury (12.4%) compared with their urban peers (6.3%).[19] Deaths among children were driven primarily by accidents and other injuries, including motor vehicle accidents, drowning, fire, suffocation, firearm injuries, and poisoning. Rural children's mortality rates associated with motor vehicle accidents were twice as high (3.1%) as urban child mortality rates (1.5%), and motor vehicle accidents were the leading cause of death among children aged 5 to 13 years. A study conducted in Wisconsin found that teenagers aged 15 to 19 years had the highest rate of pediatric ambulance runs, with motor vehicle accidents representing the most common type of injury.[20]

Rural-residing children experience higher suicide mortality than children living in urban areas.[21] During the coronavirus disease 2019 (COVID-19) pandemic, rural pediatric emergency department visits and subsequent hospitalizations for suicide or self-harm increased significantly, highlighting a pressing need to find ways to meet the behavioral health needs of rural pediatric populations.[21]

Rural Emergency Medical Service Pediatric Capabilities

Children represented a modest share of all EMS responses (6.3% of 911 responses in 2019,[22] 13% of EMS transports from 1997 to 2000[23]). Based on data from the 1997 to 2000 National Hospital Ambulatory Medical Care Survey, children's annual EMS utilization rates were 26 EMS visits per 1,000 children compared with 66 EMS visits per 1,000 adults ($P<.001$).[23] Approximately two-thirds (62%) of pediatric patients were transported because of injury or poisoning.[23]

EMS agencies face unique challenges when responding to pediatric calls, which may lead to poorer quality of care compared with adults. For example, EMS providers may lack training or have limited opportunity to practice skills on pediatric patients.[24–26] A statewide study of pediatric behavioral health-related EMS encounters in Florida found that 25% of calls were related to substance use and that EMS services were ill equipped to care for pediatric patients, particularly in areas where limited psychiatric services were available.[27] Another study found Tribal EMS services generally faced higher than average ratios of ambulance to service populations and often lacked medical directors and the ability to provide pediatric continuing education.[28] In addition, ambulances may lack equipment in the sizes optimal for serving pediatric patients.[26] These challenges may be worse among rural EMS providers with lower volume, particularly in EDs.

Ambulance Deserts and Pediatric Populations

Given children's vulnerability to accidents and sudden illnesses, living in rural areas–particularly ADs—may present unique risks for children. In an AD, where access to timely emergency medical care is limited, the inability to swiftly respond to these emergencies significantly increases the risk of adverse outcomes including morbidity and mortality. Without prompt access to emergency medical care, even minor incidents can escalate into life-threatening situations. Prolonged response times may lead to poorer outcomes for children in acute medical crises, such as severe allergic reactions, respiratory distress, or traumatic injuries.

To address causes and solutions to rural ADs it is critical to understand adverse social determinants of health affecting children. The authors addressed the socioeconomic characteristics and geographic location of pediatric populations living in ADs within 8 states within the continental United States: Northeast (Vermont and Maine), South (Texas, North Carolina), West (Montana, New Mexico) and the Midwest (Indiana, Missouri).[1] Census block-level AD data were obtained from the Maine Rural Health Research Center. The socioeconomic characteristics of children living in ADs were obtained from the 2016 to 2020 American Community Survey 5-year estimates and included age, gender, race, education levels, employment status, federal poverty levels (FPLs), geographic location, and insurance status.[29] Rural urban continuum codes were used to identify ADs falling within rural and urban counties,[30] while the 2019 rural urban commuting area (RUCA) codes were used to identify ADs within each of the 4 categories of urban, large rural, small rural, and isolated small rural census tracts.[31,32] Ambulance locations and deserts were identified and mapped using the ArcGIS Desktop ArcMap version 10.8.1.[33]

Using these research methods, pediatric risk factors associated with living in ADs included: living in more remote rural locations, older pediatric populations (particularly teenagers aged 15 to 17 years), being Native American, living in high poverty areas, and living in areas with high uninsurance rates. The fact that teenagers aged 15 to 19 years experienced among the highest mortality rates for motor vehicle crashes[20] and the fact that they also face among the highest odds of living in ADs, accentuates the need to address these gaps in acute care services. This same study documented that more remote rural locations tended to have higher rates of pediatric ambulance runs, an alarming statistic given that the AD study has documented that pediatric populations living in more remote rural locations are 8 times more likely to live in ADs.

The authors documented significant variation in racial and ethnic disparities across the states, illustrated by relatively high concentrations of Hispanic populations living in ADs in Texas and New Mexico. Native American populations were also at greater risk of living in ADs and were more likely to live in rural areas. Thus, identifying factors that place pediatric minority populations at risk for accessing ambulance services, and integrating and supporting Tribal EMS services within the overall network of ambulance services throughout the states are important policy issues that state EMS offices will need to consider.

Of concern to the sustainability of rural ambulance services is that rural pediatric populations are more likely to refuse transport to an emergency department, particularly among calls taken by Tribal EMS agencies.[22] In order to bill for services, current reimbursement policies require that ambulance services transport patients to an ED. Reasons underlying transport refusals, and the impact on patient safety and the financial sustainability of rural ambulance services warrant further study.

SUMMARY

Gaps in the provision of ambulance services are placing children at risk of adverse health outcomes associated with acute illness or injury, particularly in remote rural locations. Given that rural pediatric populations tend to be more socially vulnerable than urban populations, are more likely to live in health professional shortage areas and face higher mortality and morbidity risks associated with illness or injury than their urban peers,[1] rural ambulance services capable of treating vulnerable pediatric populations are of critical importance. In many remote rural areas throughout the United States, ambulance staff are often the first and only point of care and are an important safety net for areas with high concentrations of uninsured rural populations.[34] Finding ways to support ambulance service safety nets in impoverished remote rural locations throughout the United States and ensure that ambulance crews have the proper training to care for pediatric populations should be a high priority among state and federal policy makers.

Promoting reforms that ensure access to timely ambulance services among children, including minority populations living in rural areas, as well as alternative models that support the financial viability of rural EMS while enabling access to coordinated primary and emergent care is an important area of policy concern. Aside from strategies to address workforce shortages by incentivizing health care providers to serve in rural areas,[35] proposed (rural) solutions to address social determinants of health, acute behavioral health issues, and acute chronic conditions such as asthma[36] and seizures[37] include telehealth[17] and expanding EMS-based services in the community. The business case for reimbursing EMS providers caring for patients outside the walls of a health care facility is slowly gaining momentum within emerging models of EMS services known as community paramedicine or mobile integrated health (MIH).[27,38,39]

Low volume issues and the high costs associated with variable (eg, staff training, standby/on call hours) and fixed (eg, ambulance and equipment) costs imply that rural ambulance services struggle to break even based on the traditional reimbursement model of bringing patients to the hospital or the emergency department. Other rural providers, including critical access hospitals facing similar issues have advocated and received cost-based reimbursement,[40,41] a concept that policymakers interested in sustaining and filling rural ambulance coverage gaps have been exploring.

In closing, in lieu of badly needed federal and state level reforms, communities interested in supporting the provision of EMS services have been doing so at a grassroots level. To address the need to support communities in their strategic planning efforts, the Maine Rural Health Action Network has developed a toolkit to help communities identify the level of services that they can support using a process referred to as informed community self-determination (ICSD).[42] This process enables rural community members to work with a team of ICSD guides to evaluate their existing service(s), identify issues, as well as resources and solutions, and guide communities toward developing the type of ambulance service that meets their needs. While EMS providers have traditionally relied on grassroots efforts to organize and support their services, documenting the prevalence of ambulance deserts throughout the United States and the extent to which vulnerable populations, such as children, are living in them, has provided policymakers with the evidence needed to propose much needed policy reforms that will help ensure access to ambulance services.

CLINICS CARE POINTS

- ADs lead to increased pediatric morbidity and mortality.
- Rural communities are less likely to have the financial and personnel resources to support a robust EMS system.
- Rural EMS systems are challenged by a lack of expertise in caring for pediatric emergencies.

- A collaborative system of care that integrates regional pediatric experts with rural EMS programs using simulation training and telemedicine could help bridge the current AD gap.

FUNDING

This work was supported by the Federal Office of Rural Health Policy (FORHP), Health Resources and Services Administration (HRSA), Grant CA#U1CRH03716, Rural Health Research Center Cooperative Agreement to the Maine Rural Health Research Center.The information, conclusions and opinions expressed are those of the authors and no endorsement by FORHP, HRSA, or HHS is intended or should be inferred.

REFERENCES

1. Jonk Y, O'Connor H, DeAngelis T, et al. Disparities in accessing ambulance services: variations by state and across US census regions. Presented at: National Rural Health Association Annual Meeting; May 9 2024; New Orleans, Louisiana.
2. Jonk Y, Milkowski C, Croll Z, Pearson K. Ambulance Deserts: Geographic Disparities in the Provision of Ambulance Services [Chartbook]. University of Southern Maine, Muskie School, Maine Rural Health Research Center; 2023.
3. Bolton A. Rural ambulance services are in jeopardy as volunteers age and expenses mount. Kaiser Health News. 2021. Available at: https://khn.org/news/article/rural-ambulance-services-are-in-jeopardy-as-volunteers-age-and-expenses-mount/.
4. Dean J. Costs, volunteer demands strain rural ambulance services. Cornell University; 2022. Available at: https://news.cornell.edu/stories/2022/04/costs-volunteer-demands-strain-rural-ambulance-services.
5. Gau D, Busch F. Rural EMS 'at a critical point': southwest Minn. agencies struggling to find enough EMTs to cover shifts. Marshall Independent Online News; 2022. Available at: https://www.marshallindependent.com/news/local-news/2022/04/rural-ems-at-a-critical-point/.
6. Federal Interagency Committee on Emergency Medical Services. 2011 National EMS Assessment. US Department of Transportation, National Highway Traffic Safety Administration, DOT HS 811 723, Washington, DC, 2012.
7. Calams S. Private vs. public ambulance services: What's the difference? EMS News 2017. Available at: https://www.ems1.com/private-public-dispute/articles/private-vs-public-ambulance-services-whats-the-difference-WTgJNJgR4KIljlV9/.
8. National Association of State EMS Officials, 2020 National emergency medical services assessment. NASEMSO, Available at: https://nasemso.org/wp-content/uploads/2020-National-EMS-Assessment_Reduced-File-Size.pdf, (Accessed 21 March 2024), 2020.
9. Shah MN. The formation of the emergency medical services system. Am J Publ Health 2006;96(3):414–23.
10. NEMSAC Advisory, National EMS Advisory Council Committee report and advisory, Available at: https://www.ems.gov/assets/NEMSAC_Final_Advisory_EMS_System_Funding_Reimbursement.pdf. (Accessed 21 March 2024).
11. Jonk Y, Wingrove G, Nudell N, et al. A consensus panel approach to estimating the start-up and annual service costs for rural ambulance agencies. Policy Brief 2023.
12. MacKinney AC, Mueller KJ, Coburn AF, et al. Characteristics and challenges of rural ambulance agencies – a brief review and policy considerations. Rural Policy Research Institute. Available at: https://rupri.org/wp-content/uploads/Characteristics-and-Challenges-of-Rural-Ambulance-Agencies-January-2021.pdf.

13. National Advisory Committee on Rural Health and Human Services, Access to emergency medical services in rural communities: policy brief and recommendations to the Secretary, Available at: https://www.hrsa.gov/sites/default/files/hrsa/advisory-committees/rural/access-to-ems-rural-communities.pdf. (Accessed 21 March 2024).
14. Probst JC, Barker JC, Enders A, et al. Current state of child health in rural america: how context shapes children's health. J Rural Health 2018;34(Suppl 1):s3–12.
15. What Is shortage designation? Health Resources & Services Administration. Available at: https://bhw.hrsa.gov/workforce-shortage-areas/shortage-designation#hpsas. Accessed March 27, 2024.
16. Theriault H, Bridge G. Oral health equity for rural communities: where are we now and where can we go from here? Br Dent J 2023;235(2):99–102.
17. Childrens Health Fund. 15 million kids in health care deserts: can telehealth make a difference? Samsung Innovation Center at Children's Health Fund. Available at: https://www.childrenshealthfund.org/wp-content/uploads/2016/12/CHF_Health-Care-Deserts.pdf. Accessed March 21, 2024.
18. Pullmann MD, VanHooser S, Hoffman C, et al. Barriers to and supports of family participation in a rural system of care for children with serious emotional problems. Community Ment Health J 2010;46(3):211–20.
19. Garnett M, Spencer M, Hedegaard H. Urban-rural differences in unintentional injury death rates among children aged 0–17 years: United States, 2018–2019: NCHS Data Brief # 421. US DHHS, Centers for Disease Control and Prevention. Available at: https://www.cdc.gov/nchs/data/databriefs/db421.pdf. Accessed March 21, 2024.
20. Pediatric ambulance runs: facts and trends. Wisconsin Office of Preparedness and Emergency Health Care. Available at: https://www.dhs.wisconsin.gov/publications/p02508.pdf. Accessed March 28, 2024.
21. Arakelyan M, Emond JA, Leyenaar JK. Suicide and self-harm in youth presenting to a US rural hospital during COVID-19. Hosp Pediatr 2022;12(10):e336–42.
22. Ward C, Zhang A, Brown K, et al. National characteristics of non-transported children by emergency medical services in the United States. Prehosp Emerg Care 2022;26(4):537–46.
23. Shah MN, Cushman JT, Davis CO, et al. The epidemiology of emergency medical services use by children: an analysis of the National Hospital Ambulatory Medical Care Survey. Prehosp Emerg Care 2008;12(3):269–76.
24. Hansen M, Loker W, Warden C. Geospatial analysis of pediatric EMS run density and endotracheal intubation. West J Emerg Med 2016;17(5):656–61.
25. Stevens SL, Alexander JL. The impact of training and experience on EMS providers' feelings toward pediatric emergencies in a rural state. Pediatr Emerg Care 2005;21(1):12–7.
26. Ross SW, Campion E, Jensen AR, et al. Prehospital and emergency department pediatric readiness for injured children: a statement from the American College of Surgeons Committee on Trauma Emergency Medical Services Committee. J Trauma Acute Care Surg 2023;95(2):e6–10.
27. Fishe JN, Lynch S. Pediatric behavioral health-related EMS encounters: a statewide analysis. Prehosp Emerg Care 2019;23(5):654–62.
28. Genovesi AL, Hastings B, Edgerton EA, et al. Pediatric emergency care capabilities of Indian Health Service emergency medical service agencies serving American Indians/Alaska Natives in rural and frontier areas. Rural Rem Health 2014;14(2):2688.

29. American Community Survey (ACS). United States Census Bureau. Available at: https://www.census.gov/programs-surveys/acs. Accessed June 22, 2022.
30. US Department of Agriculture ERS. 2023 rural-urban continuum codes. 2024. Available at: https://www.ers.usda.gov/data-products/rural-urban-continuum-codes/. Accessed May 14, 2024.
31. 2010 rural-urban commuting area codes, Available at: https://www.ers.usda.gov/data-products/rural-urban-commuting-area-codes/. (Accessed 27 March 2024).
32. Using RUCA data, Available at: https://depts.washington.edu/uwruca/ruca-uses.php. (Accessed 21 March 2024).
33. ArcGIS desktop. Environmental Systems Research Institute (ESRI), Available at: https://www.esri.com/en-us/arcgis/products/arcgis-desktop/overview. (Accessed 22 June 2024).
34. King N, Pigman M, Huling S, Hanson B. EMS services in rural America: Challenges and Opportunities: A Policy Brief. National Rural Health Association. Available at: https://www.ruralhealth.us/NRHA/media/Emerge_NRHA/Advocacy/Policy%20documents/05-11-18-NRHA-Policy-EMS.pdf. Accessed March 21, 2024.
35. Davis CS, Meyers P, Bazemore AW, et al. Impact of service-based student loan repayment program on the primary care workforce. Ann Fam Med 2023;21(4):327–31.
36. Estrada RD, Ownby DR. Rural asthma: current understanding of prevalence, patterns, and interventions for children and adolescents. Curr Allergy Asthma Rep 2017;17(6):37.
37. Firnberg MT, Lerner EB, Nan N, et al. National variation in EMS response and antiepileptic medication administration for children with seizures in the prehospital setting. West J Emerg Med 2023;24(4):805–13.
38. Bennett KJ, Yuen MW, Merrell MA. Community paramedicine applied in a rural community. J Rural Health 2018;34(Suppl 1):s39–47.
39. Mobile Integrated Healthcare–Community Paramedicine (MIH-CP) National Association of Emergency Medical Technicians (NAEMT). 2024. Available at: https://www.naemt.org/resources/mih-cp#:~:text=Mobile%20Integrated%20Healthcare%E2%80%93Community%20Paramedicine,out%2Dof%2Dhospital%20environment. Accessed March 28, 2024.
40. Rural Health Information Hub, Critical access hospitals (CAHs), Available at: https://www.ruralhealthinfo.org/topics/critical-access-hospitals. (Accessed 28 March 2024).
41. MedPAC, Critical access hospitals payment system, Available at: https://www.medpac.gov/wp-content/uploads/2022/10/MedPAC_Payment_Basics_23_CAH_FINAL_SEC.pdf, (Accessed 28 March 2024), 2023.
42. McGinnis K, Wingrove G. Template for emergency medical services informed community self determination (ICSD). Wisconsin Ambulance Agency Assessment.

Reimagining Neonatal Follow-Up

An Equitable Model of Care Emphasizing Family and Child Function

Paige Terrien Church, MD[a,*], Rudaina Banihani, MD[b],
Jonathan Samuel Litt, MD[a], Michael Msall, MD[c]

KEYWORDS

- Neonatal follow-up • Health care equity • Hybrid care • Neonatal outcomes
- Behavioral phenotype of prematurity

KEY POINTS

- Despite advances in neonatal intensive care units care, neonatal follow-up programs exhibit significant variability in staffing, care provision, and resource allocation.
- Key to behavioral phenotypes is the developmental principle that development is not binary but rather a fluid process that does not always happen in a smooth arc but can occur in fits and bursts.
- Rigid models of follow-up care are out of date with the evidence and potentially not delivering effective or cost-efficient care.

BACKGROUND

Neonatal Follow-up History

The initial goal of neonatal follow-up (NFU) was to assess outcomes resulting from care in neonatal intensive care units (NICUs), which were newly established, focusing on neonates rather than all pediatric patients.[1] These outcomes encompassed the identification of the potential sequelae of care, particularly in neonates who survived into the toddler period and exhibited disabling conditions such as cerebral palsy (CP), visual/hearing disability, or cognitive impairment.[2] Surveillance for such outcomes served as a quality check on new interventions, increases that might necessitate an evaluation of care efficacy. For years, as care in the NICU rapidly evolved and

[a] Department of Neonatology, Beth Israel Deaconess Medical Center, 330 Brookline Avenue, Rose 334, Boston, MA 02215, USA; [b] Department of Neonatology, Sunnybrook Health Sciences Centre, 1875 Bayview Avenue, Toronto, Ontario M5N 3T5, Canada; [c] Department of Pediatrics, Comer Children's Hospital, 5721 South Maryland Avenue, Chicago, IL 60637, USA
* Corresponding author.
E-mail address: pchurch1@bidmc.harvard.edu

Pediatr Clin N Am 72 (2025) 93–109
https://doi.org/10.1016/j.pcl.2024.07.027 **pediatric.theclinics.com**

new practices were implemented, these outcomes were evaluated with the contemporary epoch of care in mind.[2–4] However, recent trends indicate a shift toward more standardized and less fluctuant care, resulting in greater stability in the prevalence of these short-term outcomes.[5]

Furthermore, long-term, older adolescent and adult studies have demonstrated important, unmeasured outcomes around function and quality of life.[6] These studies have called into question the significance and relevance of the initial short-term measures of outcome.[7] Significantly, parents have questioned the importance of the reported toddler outcomes, articulating a need for outcomes related to function, such as a child's feeding abilities, sleeping regulation, hospitalizations, future behavioral skills, and progress in adaptive skills essential for learning with peers in preschool and school learning environments.[8]

As NICU care evolved, so too did NFU programs and the clinical expertise of caring for preterm infants as they grow. The initial goals for programs on outcomes documentation of major motor, neurosensory, and cognitive disability shifted toward developing expertise in identification and proactive intervention for a wider spectrum of health, neurodevelopmental, and behavior disorders. The Bayley Scales of Infant Development (BSID)—the most commonly used assessment tool in NDU—has been proven to have limited predictive accuracy for significant challenges[9,10] at older ages. However, other assessments have been identified that are highly accurate for the identification of specific outcomes, such as CP[11] and sensorineural hearing loss.[12] Children with ASD, once not diagnosed until 3 or 4 years of age at the earliest, are now being identified in the toddler period, enabling specific interventions to be initiated.[13] Similarly, children with CP, once not diagnosed until 2 years of age, are now being identified as early as 3 months of age, and targeted intervention is initiated.[14] The benefits of early intervention have also been well demonstrated, particularly with outcomes such as autism spectrum disorder (ASD),[13]CP,[14] sensorineural hearing loss,[12] and developmental disabilities.[15] Long-standing partnerships have been forged between NFU and early intervention programs,[16] and there is an increased recognition for more systematic neurodevelopmental surveillance and proactive interventions to optimize functioning, school readiness, and academic achievement.

CHALLENGES IN NEONATAL FOLLOW-UP

Despite advances in NICU care, NFU programs exhibit significant variability in staffing, care provision, and resource allocation.[17,18] A recent assessment in the United States, over a decade old, demonstrated tremendous variability in staffing and follow-up schedules[17] and mirrored the same pattern from a recent Canadian study.[18] Funding remains a pervasive issue,[17,18] affecting the educational experience for medical trainees, with limited guidance from certifying bodies like the American Board of Pediatrics or the Royal College of Canada in follow-up training other than to indicate its need.[19,20] Dual training in Neonatal-Perinatal Medicine and Developmental (Behavioral) Pediatrics has emerged but has challenges of additional training time, funding, and lack of mentorship. Fewer than 10 individuals are dually certified in the United States and Canada. Other dual training opportunities include Neonatal Neurology and Complex Care, which face similar obstacles.

Another long-standing challenge for NFU programs has been follow-up adherence. No-show or lost-to-follow-up rates are a consistent challenge, especially among non-English-speaking or Black families.[21] One common theme is the cost to families.[22] While Canada provides a socialized health care system, and therefore, visits for health care are free of direct cost, there is the cost of time off from work or transportation and parking. For those in the United States, copays from insurance and the above challenges compound the cost and limit attendance. Further to the cost, there is a common experience of parental trauma from the NICU experience and reigniting this trauma, returning to a health care facility with their preterm child for assessment.[23] The location for NFU programs is often in tertiary centers, located in urban areas not proximal to rural families, requiring extensive travel to attend follow-up.[22,24,25] Lastly, for those where travel is essential for NFU care, weather can pose a significant challenge for several months of the year, limiting access to needed appointments.[24]

OUTCOMES OF PRETERM CHILDREN

What has emerged from years of data collected has informed the behavioral phenotype of the preterm child.[26] This behavioral phenotype includes a spectrum of strengths and challenges across attention, behavior, regulation, and peer social skills. The common biological etiology of this behavioral phenotype after extreme prematurity is brain dysmaturation resulting from preterm birth and includes causal pathways of aberrant environmental exposures of the NICU, separation from parents, stress, and inflammation.[26–29] Encapsulating behavior patterns into these behavioral phenotypes allows greater ease of identification and earlier intervention[27] for the spectrum of attention, executive function, regulatory behaviors, and social skills that underlie school and community success. Key to behavioral phenotypes is the developmental principle that development is not binary but rather a fluid process that does not always happen in a smooth arc but can occur in fits and bursts. Rather than normal or abnormal, most development is characterized as typical or expected, variant or still within the range of expected but on the outer aspect of expected. Atypical development, including problem behavior or development, is environmentally mediated and improves with environmental modifications. Finally, there is disordered development or behavior, presenting in multiple environments and interfering with day-to-day function.[30] Key to the behavioral phenotype for the preterm is that challenges may emerge as problems and/or disorders rather than exclusively disorders.[26] Specifically, there is a wide spectrum of impacts that require attention to a whole child framework of neurodiversity.

Preterm infants exhibit notable strengths within this framework, often characterized by reported happiness and resilience. Parents frequently admire their child's survival and developmental progress aligning with expectations.[9] For each child, the challenges may ebb and flow in terms of the developmental stream impacted and age, as gaps present only when that area of the dysmature cortex is developmentally expected.[31] The presence and degree of functional impact is variable, with some unaffected, others minimally impacted, and others more impacted.[26] Generally, the more preterm the child, the more pronounced the challenge and its functional impact.[26] It is rare to have one isolated challenge; rather, they often present with a constellation of challenges.[26] It is equally important that the spectrum of these disorders do not preclude developmental progress, learning, and social success.

The minority of preterm survivors has significant morbidity characterized by disabling disorder, such as CP, vision or hearing impairment, and cognitive impairment.[2,26] The prevalence of these outcomes varies widely, ranging from 3% to 25%, contingent upon gestational age and specific diagnostic criteria.[4,26] Many preterm survivors experience minor challenges with motor skills, behavioral regulation, learning skills, language and communication, and social skills.[26] Motor challenges include visual motor discrepancies, making copying and creating images or letters difficult.[32,33] Learning to write and then writing to learn becomes challenging, as the effort is more effortful and inefficient. In some preterm children, there is an increased possibility of developmental coordination disorder presenting with persistent challenges mastering day-to-day functional motor tasks, for which practice does not improve performance.[34] Identification and specific cognitive approaches to improve function.[35] Behavioral regulation with increased attentional weakness/attention deficit disorder and executive function challenges are more common in the former preterm.[26,33] Tasks with directions in series are often inaccurately followed. Persistence in tasks can be exquisitely challenging for a preterm child, particularly for those tasks that are more difficult.[33] Emotional regulation can also be more erratic in the preterm child, with preterm children presenting with greater emotional lability.[36] Learning disabilities in reading, mathematics, and written language are more common in the former preterm and can be late to be diagnosed, exacerbating greater behavioral problems.[26,33] Much less common is intellectual disability.[26,33,37] Communication difficulties manifest across various dimensions, such as language comprehension, auditory processing, articulation, and sentence complexity.[26,33] Socially, preterm children have been described as more nomadic, preferring adults or older children over peer engagements, potentially influenced by language challenges or comorbidities such as ASD.[26,37,38] However, empirical data on ASD prevalence among preterm populations remain sparse, albeit suggestive of heightened vulnerability among extremely premature infants.[38]

Transition to school can be tumultuous as many educators are unaware of this phenotype, and identification requires discrete, specific assessment, which is costly and time-consuming.[26,39,40] Moreover, discontinuation of follow-up programs and early intervention services by the age of 3 years deprives families of ongoing support, exacerbating challenges associated with navigating the complexities of the preterm behavioral phenotype.[17,18,26] In addition, limited requirements exist for pediatric trainees or developmental-behavioral/neurodevelopmental pediatrics on the behavioral phenotype of prematurity, leaving health care practitioners ill-equipped to provide expert guidance and consultation to affected families.[19,20]

The underlying etiology of the behavioral phenotype of prematurity is the dysmaturation of the preterm brain[28,29]—the combination of epigenetics, environment, and inflammation.[28,29] For the preterm brain, development in the third and possibly the second trimester occurs in the unnatural environment of the NICU. Separated from its parent, introduced to novel environmental stimuli with sounds through air, touch, pain, and gravity, the brain develops differently.[28,29] At a genetic level, changes in gene methylation signal the brain's adaptive nature to its experience.[41,42] At a cellular level, cells are programmed to receive input. Some inputs are premature and excessive, leading to connections and pathways that may not be intended. The input is absent or minimized in others, leading to diminished connectivity.[26,28,29] Exacerbating this is the vulnerability to injury, with cells not having protective mechanisms to manage stressors such as excessive oxygen exposure, which leads to oxidative injury or inflammation.[29] At the sensory system level, the input received by the preterm infant is altered and isolated, and it has been hypothesized to contribute to future dysregulation.[42] In utero, the child experiences most sensory input in a multimodal manner; a sound is muffled through amniotic fluid, providing auditory input and associated vestibular input as the fetus startles or moves to the sound. In the NICU, however, with the confines of gravity and essential tubing, sensory inputs become isolated and splintered from the expected multimodal input.[42] The result is cellular loss, diminished cortical volume, diminished and altered connectivity, sensory dysregulation, and potentially more significant injury superimposed on this dysmaturation.[28,29,41,42]

At a developmental level, the impact of this complex interaction between the developing brain, a novel environment, and parental separation is a difference in musculature development. Historically referred to as transient abnormal neurologic signs, this describes the preterm motor pattern with extensor posturing, scapular retraction, and diminished flexural strength.[43,44] This pattern tends to improve over the first 2 years of life and, historically, has been a confounding finding with attempts to identify CP early.[45]

Additionally, the etiology of the behavioral phenotype of prematurity is also rooted in the injury to parents.[26,46] For many parents, the NICU is a foreign place with a novel language, culture, and expectations.[47,48] Parents having experienced the NICU have a greater likelihood of postnatal depression, anxiety, and posttraumatic stress, and this increased possibility is not selective for the birth parent only but affects both parents.[48,49] There is strong evidence demonstrating that parental mental health impacts the process of attachment.[50] This increased possibility of mental health challenges for parents,[48,49] combined with a child that has experienced ongoing daily dysregulation with variable sensory exposures[42] and consequently is not regulated themselves,[26,37] leads to significant potential challenges with attachment.[50]

CHANGES DRIVING CHANGE

The Pandemic and Telehealth

The pandemic with severe acute respiratory syndrome coronavirus 2, or coronavirus disease 2019 (COVID-19), presented an opportunity within the health care crisis. Before the pandemic, virtual telehealth had been mired in proprietary technology, ongoing challenges to accessibility with technology not being equitably distributed, and privacy concerns.[51] To accommodate limited access to health care during COVID-19, these challenges at a global level quickly dissolved, and virtual visits became a new normal and were implemented in NFU.[52,53] While limitations to this forum for health care were identified, benefits have persisted, particularly around accessibility for families, the opportunity for families to interact with providers without having to leave their homes, and minimizing costs for many families.[54,55] It was feasible to coordinate additional consultants on the virtual visit as this could be done from one's office rather than commuting to a mutual space for assessment.[56] Lastly, for non-English speaking families, there was the benefit of adding an interpreter online rather than the interpreter having to travel to the assessment space.[55–57] As COVID-19 has become less of a day-to-day concern, the use of virtual health has also diminished. Other challenges in addition to inconsistent implementation has been uncertainty in reimbursement depending on insurance, organization, and state/country.[57]

Family Voices

Another seismic change to NFU has been an increasingly vocal parent advisory groups that have formed partnerships with networks such as the Vermont Oxford Network and Canadian Neonatal Follow-Up Network (CNFUN), and others. Adding to this are a growing population of NICU providers who have gained experience as parents/grandparents of a child in the NICU.[58] This new generation of parents/grandparents have provided greater insight into outcomes of importance to parents and families, and the outcomes they identify do not align with those deemed important by medicine.[8,9] Rather challenges around feeding and sleeping regulation, admissions to hospital, breathing, and behavioral and school-based difficulties have been raised as outcomes that are more relevant to families.[9] These outcomes align with those deemed significant by Rosenbaum and colleagues,[59] with emphasis on "F" words; function by doing what you can, fitness for proactive health, fun by having a passion for the achievable, family and friends for support and encouragement, and a future of possibilities. Implementing protocols to better measure and reflect these important parent-identified outcomes is an ongoing goal.

Early Detection

Early identification has emerged as feasible and associated with better functional outcomes for both ASD[13] and CP.[14] In the preterm population, both conditions have an increased incidence with decreasing gestation.[3,4,26,37] For ASD, the pathway remains unchanged from that of term children, with a focus on screening for social communication and behavior skills early.[13] For the preterm child, however, with features consistent with possible ASD, a full assessment is warranted. There are no current guidelines for assessment and diagnosis. Drawing upon other populations with comorbid and potentially confounding developmental conditions, the practice of a full assessment for autism using a standardized tool, the Autism Diagnostic Observation Schedule, second edition, is recommended.[14,60] CP, however, has clear care guidelines demonstrating the feasibility of early identification with precise established tools and the benefit of early intervention.[13,45] When used in combination, neuroimaging and clinical tools of the General Movement Assessment (GMA) and Hammersmith Infant Neurological Examination (HINE) have demonstrated synergy with early identification.[11] The GMA is an observational assessment of the quality of an infant's (preterm to 20 weeks postterm) whole-body movements and has been correlated to underlying neurologic integrity. The HINE is a standardized neurologic examination of an infant between 2 and 24 months, including tone, posture, reflexes, and reactions, as well as asymmetric findings.[11,14] This shift places greater emphasis on earlier and more comprehensive NFU visits.

Flexible and Responsive Care

Lastly, harmonized care has been demonstrated to be feasible.[61] In Ontario, the centralized health care system prioritized a system of NFU that was equitable and accessible.[61,62] Identified challenges were familiar to those described for all NFU programs, including disparity in staffing and funding, inconsistent schedules, distance to care and travel, and cost with time off from work and/or parking.[61] Additionally, there was the challenge of the large geographic region of Ontario, with some families requiring flights to attend appointments and weather.[61] The Provincial Council of Maternal and Child Health (PCMCH) assembled a working group to evaluate the status of follow-up across the province and then attempt to harmonize the system. Over 3 years, the group demonstrated that while there was variability in staffing, there was a consistent commitment to the families and their children and a unifying interest in care provision closer to home.[61,62] With this, the group identified a "touchpoints" approach to care, focusing on the child's and family's developmental needs.[61] The group used this touchpoints approach to facilitate harmony in schedules. The recommendations did not mandate specific neurodevelopmental assessments but rather allowed each specific team to identify the tool that suited their individual staffing capacity and skill set.[61] A shared care model was developed with families and children having the option to have care in follow-up programs closer to home, in close collaboration with the tertiary center for support.[61,62] The more immature the child, the greater the involvement of the tertiary team, to allocate resources to those in need.[61,62]

ALTERNATIVE MODELS OF CARE

Other models of care have been proposed that have either collaborated with NFU programs or, in some settings, merged. Complex care is a field that evolved to provide medical coordination of care for children with complex medical conditions, requiring multiple subspecialty providers.[63] This medical model centers the child and family with the local pediatrician and therapy team. There are established contacts with the complex care coordination team in the subspecialty center for both parents and providers.[64] This hub-and-spoke model has allowed for better care coordination in more rural environments and minimized travel and cost to parents with focused trips, providing as much exposure to providers as needed and possible.[64] This model has also allowed local providers to be more empowered to provide the required and supported care.[63,64]

In addition, addressing parental mental health is crucial in any model of care for families navigating NICU experiences. Strategies for managing parental anxiety and depression in the NICU have encompassed parental education, involvement in day-to-day care, and counseling.[65] Evidence has demonstrated heterogeneous findings with mixed impacts on parental anxiety and depression.[65,66] One counseling approach utilizes cognitive behavioral therapy, as this has had strong evidence in generalized anxiety disorder models.[67] In this context, one is taught to examine one's thoughts and appreciate the gap between the thoughts and reality and then to learn skills to manage this gap.[67] In the NICU reality, however, most parental worries are based firmly on reality, and as such, this may account for the lack of consistent evidence. A model demonstrating early feasibility is Coached Enhanced Neonatal Transitions, which utilizes a nurse-based coaching model providing greater parental capacity and consistent contact within the health care system. It added a component of mental health support, acceptance and commitment therapy (ACT).[68] ACT teaches parents to identify and focus on their values, acknowledging their concerns but keeping them in the context of that which is important to them.[68] In doing so, the worry and anxiety are shifted from a position of focus to one of peripheral vision, present but not obscuring the view of what matters. Early evidence from this approach has demonstrated feasibility.[68]

An attempt at addressing the inequity in access to care provision of care and one that attempts to address the needs of the child and family, as well as one that continues to allow for ongoing data for quality assurance, has been described. This model of NFU has been called "E-Nurture" and includes a hybridized approach to care, with virtual and in-person visits, weaving principles from complex care models, opportunities from COVID-19 and virtual care, and the experience from PCMCH's working group.[52,61,62] This concept of "touchpoints" is critical to the schedule of visits, reflecting a concept from Dr Brazelton, describing those developmental moments that can lead to struggle or conflict within a family.[52,69] They are moments of growth for the child and family.[69] When presented as such, positive elements can be appreciated, and the steps to work forward appear more proactive.

Merging this with parental values of outcomes is critical, both clinically and for reporting and quality monitoring. Recently, the CNFUN assembled teams of those involved in follow-up and parents to identify priorities in data collection.[70] Outcomes to be collected and reported were reprioritized to include those parents deemed important, with attention to feasibility.[70] Seven domains were identified: child well-being/happiness, quality of life/function, socioemotional and behavioral outcomes, respiratory, feeding, sleeping, and caregiver mental health.[70] At the 18 to 24 month research-based data collection visit, measures were identified to measure these outcomes. While these data are important and the screeners feasible, modifications are essential in order to reap a clinical benefit. Feeding challenges are often identified early following discharge, with failure to thrive peaking at 4 months corrected age as the sucking reflex integrates.[71] Capturing a feeding challenge at 18 months is important as it adds to the body of evidence but will not provide timely intervention. Similar benefits and challenges exist with the other identified domains to measure.

OPPORTUNITY TO CREATE NEONATAL FOLLOW-UP FOR THE FUTURE

Given the limitations in NFU care delivery and the innovative research being done to address them, there is tremendous opportunity to develop and test alternative, more effective models of care. This is imperative for 3 critical reasons. First, implementing and disseminating new advances in the early detection of CP and ASD will allow earlier initiation of outcome-changing therapeutic interventions. Second, the behavioral phenotype of prematurity often presents in subtle ways, requiring specialized serial assessments not commonly used today. Third, improving longer term outcomes requires longer term supports beyond the preschool period that currently marks the scope of routine NFU.

The life course health development framework has yielded greater insight into the trajectory of a diagnosis, factors that promote resilience, and practices to promote wellness and minimize disease.[72] Jonathan Litt and colleagues[73] explored the application of the life course model of care to NFU, revealing barriers stemming from fragmented systems, outdated NFU structures, and misaligned priorities. The life course model underscores the need for care across a lifespan, starting in the NICU and transitioning to the clinic with an emphasis on the health and development of the child and family, particularly as it relates to function, delivered in an equitable and accessible way.[73] Advocating for a strengths-based approach, "working toward the 'possible,'" aims to optimize existing resources for families and the child.[73] Fundamental principles to the life course model include health development with an integrated care team, acknowledging that a longitudinal approach is needed for systems of care; the complexity of health development with an ongoing interaction of the individual and environment, thus necessitating a system of care that is nimble to the many influences; timing of care sensitive to the unfolding needs of the child and family, particularly during sensitive windows; plasticity, which describes the responsive nature of the developing individual to environmental influences better described with the language of possibility rather than "fatalism"; thriving as optimizing health offers greater opportunities for success; and harmony between family needs and goals and system structures.[71,73] An opportunity exists to merge concepts of alternative models of care, including the hybrid touchpoints approach of E-Nurture, with the life-course approach, parental priorities to allow the collection of essential outcomes in real-time, using evidence to determine the timing of administration of specific tools, therefore allowing timely intervention. This model of care is described in **Table 1**. Critical to this model of care described in **Table 1** is the understanding that this can be achieved using the local resources and with integral incorporation of the pediatrician/family physician as well as family drawing from the complex care literature,[63,64] in collaboration with NFU. Parent education is a goal throughout every stage, empowering the parent to be the expert and providing consistency and more significant equity in care delivery. Additionally, developmental screening or assessment tools were chosen for feasibility and cost, using tools freely accessible as first-line choices. While the BSID has fallen under criticism for failing to provide the information that parents need/want, it does provide a comprehensive evaluation of the child with a structured opportunity to

Table 1
Touchpoint focused follow-up schedule*

Age	Touchpoint	Mode of Visit and Objective	Tool Recommended	Staffing	Intervention
Before discharge	Preparing to transition home	In-person or virtual, pending parental preference Introduction to the team and goal of the program	Written information or in-person introduction	Any team member	Assure that virtual access is possible Review medical history for triaging
1 wk after discharge	Making a place in the family	Virtual Objectives: 1. Transition to home 2. Feeding practices 3. Sleep	Virsual feeding assessment/ questionnaire Weight measurement Edinburgh Postnatal Depression Scale	Medical/nursing Social work Psychology	Referral for feeding support Mental health resources utilized Safe sleep counseling Confirm early intervention (EI) referrals are in place Determine if additional visits or subspecialty visits are needed
4 wk after discharge	The mental health of parents	Virtual Objectives 1. Mental health screening of parents 2. Initiation of early surveillance for cerebral palsy 3. Medical follow-up 4. Feeding 5. Sleep	Edinburgh Postnatal Depression Scale Assessment of general movements (parents can provide video) Virtual feeding assessment or questionnaire Sleep hygiene	Medical/nursing Social work Psychology Therapy	Referral for mental health support Liaise with subspecialty providers Referral for EI if not done Teaching around time in prone Sleep hygiene principles reviewed Feeding principles reviewed

(*continued on next page*)

Table 1
(*continued*)

Age	Touchpoint	Mode of Visit and Objective	Tool Recommended	Staffing	Intervention
4 mo	Roles established in the family and rituals needed	In-person/virtual possible Objectives 1. Examination for early signs of cerebral palsy 2. Medical follow-up/ growth parameters 3. Feeding and introduction of solids	Assessment of general movements HINE Feeding surveillance Sleep surveillance	Medical/nursing Therapy	Tummy time Advance to solids reviewed (expected in future) Sleep hygiene
8 mo	Emerging independence	In-person/virtual possible Objectives 1. Examination for early signs of CP 2. Medical follow-up/ growth 3. Feeding and solids 4. Emerging independence safety and transition postures	HINE Feeding surveillance Sleep surveillance	Medical/nursing Therapy	Transition postures reviewed. Feeding strategies with the shift from feeding to eating Sleep hygiene
12 mo	Standing and walking	Virtual or in-person Objectives 1. Assessment of motor skills 2. Introduction to discipline with newly independent infant 3. Sleep hygiene. 4. Feeding	HINE Warner Initial Developmental Evaluation of Adaptive and Functional Skills (WIDEA-FS) Survey of Well-being in Youth and Children (SWYC)	Medical/nursing Therapy	Coaching on pulling to stand/walking. Behavior management strategies Referral for structured playgroup or daycare interaction

18 mo	Independence and limit setting	In-person Objectives 1. Developmental assessment of learning, language, and motor skills 2. Surveillance for social and behavioral skills 3. Data collection for reporting, if applicable (should include measures of well-being, function, feeding, and sleeping)	Comprehensive developmental assessment (Bayley Scales of Infant Development offers historical and international reference, Mullen) SWYC WIDEA-FS	Therapy Psychology Medical/nursing	Referral for further evaluation of Autism if concerns Daycare or playgroup Behavior management strategies Speech and language strategies reviewed
36 mo	Preschooler, an emerging sense of self	Virtual or in-person Objectives 1. Developmental assessment of learning, language skills 2. Surveillance for social communication skills 3. Behavior Surveillance 4. Preparation for school	SWYC +/– more in-depth assessment as indicated with Bayley Scales or Mullen	Therapy Psychology Medical/nursing	Referral for daycare playgroup or preschool Behavior management

(*continued on next page*)

Table 1
(*continued*)

Age	Touchpoint	Mode of Visit and Objective	Tool Recommended	Staffing	Intervention
4–5 y	Neighbor—community growing for child	Virtual screen: in-person as indicated Objectives 1. Surveillance of skills to transition to school 2. Behavior and self-regulation	SWYC Canadian Pediatric Society, Preschool/ Kindergarten Teacher questionnaire	Medical/nursing Therapy	Referral for therapy as indicated Encourage group activities Public school is funded and available based on corrected age
7–8 y	Learning skills	Virtual screen: in-person as indicated Objectives: 1. Identification of learning differences 2. Behavior screening	SWYC Canadian Pediatric Society, Preschool/ Kindergarten Teacher questionnaire Vanderbilt ADHD Diagnostic Rating Scale If indicated, a tool for screening learning abilities: Kaufman Brief Intelligence Test Kaufman Test of Educational Achievement	Medical/nursing Psychology Therapy	Collaborate with local school board to share results and work to achieve necessary learning provisions Behavioral management Specific to attention and impulsivity Collaborate with the primary physician for possible ADHD pharmacotherapy

*Key to this model is awareness of the behavioral phenotype of prematurity and diligence with screening for the above touchpoints, with intervention provided. Children may be identified at any stage along this trajectory as having a significant neurodevelopmental condition, including CP, autism, or deafness. These children benefit from specific early identification to enhance opportunities to acquire function. Referral to specific therapeutic interventions is beyond the scope of this article, but it includes referral to appropriate subspecialty medical providers as well as therapy. However, these referrals and interventions do not preclude them from ongoing surveillance and screening for aspects of the behavioral phenotype of prematurity.

evaluate skills.[10] It also provides essential historical references and comparability, allowing programs to evaluate the quality of their care and categorize a child's skills.[10]

SUMMARY

NFU has grown and developed like the babies it has followed. It has morphed from a clinic structured for surveillance on outcome metrics to providing data identification and intervention to one working to reflect the outcomes that matter to parents.[1,2,9,70,72] Ongoing challenges with lack of follow-up training, inconsistent provision of care, and inequitable service allocation are critical barriers to effective, family-focused care.[17–20] Rigid models of follow-up care are out-of-date with the evidence and potentially not delivering effective or cost-efficient care. A hybrid model of care, with creative collaboration with local community resources and access to expertise in the behavioral phenotype of prematurity, can be developed specifically for each community resource and tailored to geography. Consistency in care can be achieved by espousing the model of touchpoints for care visits, informed by parental feedback and evidence, and emphasizing parents' education of their children through collaboration with local online resources and tertiary centers. Our overall emphasis is on collaboration for thriving, functioning, and participation. In this way, we can optimize longer term child health, developmental and functional outcomes, and parental well-being.

CLINICS CARE POINTS

- Most preterm infants survive without significant disability.
- Many, however, will have 'minor' challenges with various aspects of their development, including moving, regulating behavior, learning, communication and language, and social skills. Often, there are multiple areas of challenge amidst other areas of strengths.
- The pattern specific to preterm survivors has been referred to as the behaivoral phenotype of prematurity.
- Neonatal follow-up has evolved from one of surveillance to one of early identification and intervention, focusing on those outcomes identified as important by parents.
- Challenges persist around staffing, funding, and training with results in inconsistent and inequitable care.
- Rigid models of care perpetuate the challenges. Focusing on touchpoints and working with local resources to provide care can alleviate some challenges with care provision.

DISCLOSURE

The authors have no commercial or financial conflicts of interest to disclose.

REFERENCES

1. Needleman H. Introduction. In: Needleman H, Jackson BJ, editors. Follow-up for NICU graduates: promoting positive developmental and behavioral outcomes for at-risk infants. Cham, Switzerland: Springer; 2018.
2. Vohr BR, Wright LL, Dusick AM, et al. Neurodevelopmental and Functional Outcomes of Extremely Low Birth Weight Infants in the National Institute of Child Health and Human Development Neonatal Research Network, 1993-1994. Pediatrics 2000;105(6):1216–26.

3. Lemons JA, Bauer CR, Oh W, et al. Very Low Birth Weight Outcomes of the National Institute of Child Health and Human Development Neonatal Research Network, January 1995 Through December 1996. Pediatrics 2001;107(1):e1.
4. Synnes A, Luu TM, Moddemann D, et al. Determinants of developmental outcomes in a very preterm Canadian cohort. ADC Fetal Neonatal Ed 2017;102: F235–43.
5. Stoll BJ, Hansen NI, Bell EF, et al. Trends in Care Practices, Morbidity, and Mortality of Extremely Preterm Neonates, 1993-2012. JAMA 2015;314(10):1039–51.
6. Mendonca M, Bilgin A, Wolke D. Association of Preterm Birth and Low Birth Weight With Romantic Partnership, Sexual Intercourse, and Parenthood in Adulthood. JAMA Netw Open 2019;2(7):e196961. https://doi.org/10.1001/jamanetworkopen.2019.6961.
7. McCormack MC, Litt JS. The Outcomes of Very Preterm Infants: Is It Time to Ask Different Questions. Pediatrics 2017;139(1):e20161694. https://doi.org/10.1542/peds.2016-1694.
8. Staub K, Baardsnes J, Hebert N, et al. Our child is not just a gestational age. A first-hand account of what parents want and need to know before premature birth. Acta Paediatr 2014;103:1035–8.
9. Jaworski M, Janvier A, Lefebvre F, et al. Parental Perspectives Regarding Outcomes of Very Preterm Infants: Toward a Balanced Approach. J Pediatr 2018; 200:58–63.
10. Alyward GP. Issues in Neurodevelopmental Testing of Infants Born Prematurely: The Bayley Scales of Infant Development Third Edition and Other Tools. In: Needleman H, Jackson BJ, editors. Follow-up for NICU graduates: promoting positive developmental and behavioral outcomes for at-risk infants. Cham, Switzerland: Springer; 2018.
11. Morgan C, Romeo DM, Choma O, et al. The Pooled Diagnostic Accuracy of Neuroimaging, General Movements, and Neurological Examination for Diagnosing Cerebral Palsy Early in High-Risk Infants: A Case Control Study. J Clin Med 2019;8:1879.
12. Wroblewska-Seniuk K, Dabrowski P, Szyfter W, et al. Universal newborn hearing screening: methods, results, obstacles, and benefits. Pediatr Res 2017;81: 415–22.
13. Hyman SL, Levy SE, Myers SM, et al. Identification, Evaluation, and Management of Children with Autism Spectrum Disorder. Pediatrics 2020;145(1):e20193447.
14. Morgan C, Fetters L, Adde L, et al. Early Intervention for Children Aged 0 to 2 Years With or at High Risk of Cerebral Palsy: International Clinical Practice Guideline Based on Systematic Reviews. JAMA Pediatr 2021;175(8):846–58.
15. Shonkoff JP, Hauser-Cram P. Early Intervention for Disabled Infants and Their Families: A Quantitative Analysis. Pediatrics 1987;80(5):650–8.
16. Miller K. Early Intervention for NICU Graduates. In: Needleman H, Jackson BJ, editors. Follow-up for NICU graduates: promoting positive developmental and behavioral outcomes for at-risk infants. Cham, Switzerland: Springer; 2018.
17. Kuppula VS, Tabangin M, Haberman B, et al. Current state of high-risk infant follow-up care in the United States: results of a national survey of academic follow-up programs. J Perinatol 2012;32:293–8.
18. Albahli F, Church P, Ballantyne M, et al. Neonatal follow-up programs in Canada: A national survey. Paediatr Child Health 2021;26(1):246–51.
19. ACGME program requirements for graduate medical education in neonatal-perinatal medicine.

20. Royal College of Physicians and Surgeons of Canada. Neonatal-perinatal medicine training experiences 2021.
21. Fraiman YS, Edwards EM, Horbar JD, et al. Racial Inequity in High-Risk Infant Follow-Up Among Extremely Low Birth Weight Infants. Pediatrics 2023;151(2): e2022057865.
22. Ballantyne M, Stevens B, Guttmann A, et al. Maternal and infant predictors of attendance at Neonatal Follow-Up programmes. Child Care Health Dev 2014; 40(2):250–8.
23. Greene MM, Rossman B, Patra K, et al. Depression, Anxiety, and Perinatal-Specific Posttraumatic Distress in Mothers of Very Low Birth Weight Infants in the Neonatal Intensive Care Unit. J Dev Behav Pediatr 2015;36:362–70.
24. Ballantyne M, Benzies K, Rosenbaum P, et al. Mothers' and health care providers' perspectives of the barriers and facilitators to attendance at Canadian neonatal follow-up programs. Child Care Health Dev 2015;41(5):722–33.
25. Cox E, Awe M, Sabu S, et al. Does greater distance from the hospital exacerbate socioeconomic barriers to neonatal intensive care unit clinic attendance. J Rural Med 2023;18(2):55–61. Difficulty with attendance for rural families.
26. Church PT, Banihani R, Luther M, et al. Premature Infants: The Behavioral Phenotype of the Preterm Survivor. In: Needleman H, Jackson BJ, editors. Follow-up for NICU graduates: promoting positive developmental and behavioral outcomes for at-risk infants. Cham, Switzerland: Springer; 2018.
27. Hodapp RM, Fidler DJ. Special Education and Genetics: Connections for the 21st Century. J Spec Educ 1999;33(3):130–7.
28. Back SA, Miller SP. Brain Injury in Premature Neonates: A Primary Cerebral Dysmaturation Disorder? Ann Neurol 2014;45:469–86.
29. Inder TE, Volpe JJ, Anderson PJ. Defining the Neurologic Consequences of Preterm Birth. NEJM 2023;389(5):441–53.
30. Wolraich ML, Felice ME, Drotar D, editors. The classification of child and adolescent mental diagnoses in primary care. Diagnostic and statistical manual for primary care (DSM-PC) child and adolescent version. Elk Grove Village (IL): American Academy of Pediatrics; 1996.
31. Luciana M. Cognitive development in children born preterm: Implications for theories of brain plasticity following early injury. Dev Psychopathol 2003;15:1017–47.
32. Geldof CJA, van Wassenaer AG, de Kieviet JF, et al. Visual perception and visual-motor integration in very preterm and/or very low birth weight children: A meta-analysis. Res Dev Dis 2012;33(2):726–36.
33. Pascoe L, Burnett A, Anderson PJ. Cognitive and academic outcomes of children born extremely preterm. Sem Perinatol 2021;45(8):151480.
34. Bolk J, Farooqi A, Hafstrom M, et al. Developmental Coordination Disorder and Its Association With Developmental Comorbidities at 6.5 Years In Apparently Healthy Children Born Extremely Preterm. JAMA Pediatr 2018;172(8):765–74.
35. Izadi-Najafabadi S, Rinat S, Zwicker JG. Brain functional connectivity in children with developmental coordination disorder following rehabilitation intervention. Pediatr Res 2022;91:1459–68.
36. Olsen JE, Lee KJ, Spittle A, et al, members of the Victorian Infant Collaborative Study Group. The casual effect of being born extremely preterm or extremely low birthweight on neurodevelopment and social emotional development at 2 years. Acta Paediatr 2022;111:107–14.
37. Johnson S, Marlow N. Early and long-term outcome of infants born extremely preterm. Arch Dis Child 2017;102:97–102.

38. Agrawal S, Rao SC, Bulsara MK, et al. Prevalence of Autism Spectrum Disorder in Preterm Infants: A Meta-analysis. Pediatrics 2018;142(3):e20180134.
39. Church PT, Cavanagh A, Lee SK, et al. Academic challenges for the preterm infant: Parent and educators' perspectives. Early Human Dev 2019;128:1–5.
40. Johnson S, Gilmore C, Gallimore I, et al. The long-term consequences of preterm birth: what do teachers know? Dev Med Child Neurol 2015;57(6):571–7.
41. Wheater EN, Galdi P, McCartney DL, et al. DNA methylation in relation to gestational age and brain dysmaturation in preterm infants. Brain Comm 2022;4(2): fcac056.
42. Lickliter R. The Integrated Development of Sensory Organization. Clin Perinatol 2011;38:591–603.
43. Drillien CM. Abnormal Neurological Signs in the First Year of Life in Low-birthweight Infants: Possible Prognostic Significance. Dev Med Child Neurol 1972;14:575–84.
44. Church PT, Luther M, Asztalos E. The Perfect Storm: The High Prevalence Low Severity Outcomes of the Preterm Survivor. Curr Ped Rev 2012;8(2):142–51.
45. Novak I, Morgan C, Adde L, et al. Early, Accurate Diagnosis in Cerebral Palsy: Advances in Diagnosis and Treatment. JAMA Pediatr 2017;171(9):897–907.
46. Caporali C, Pisoni C, Gasparini L, et al. A global perspective on parental stress in the neonatal intensive care unit: a meta-analytical study. J Perinatol 2020;40(12): 1739–52.
47. Church PT, Dahan M, Rule A, et al. NICU Language, Everyday Ethics, and Giving Better News: Optimizing Discussions about Disability with Families. Children 2024;11(2):242.
48. Jimenez-Palomares M, Fernandez-Rejano M, Garrido-Aridla EM, et al. The Impact of a Preterm Baby Arrival in a Family: A Descriptive Cross-Sectional Pilot Study. J Clin Med 2021;10:4494.
49. Ionio C, Colombo C, Brazzoduro V, et al. Mothers and Fathers in NICU: The Impact of Preterm Birth on Parental Distress. EJOP 2016;12(4):604–21.
50. Pisoni C, Garofoli F, Tzialla C, et al. Risk and protective factors in maternal-fetal attachment development. Early Human Dev 2014;90:S45–6.
51. Sares NS, Langkamp DL. Telehealth in Developmental-Behavioral Pediatrics. J Dev Beh Peds 2012;33(8):656–65.
52. Church PT, Banihani R, Watson J, et al. The E-Nurture Project: A Hybrid Virtual Neonatal Follow Up Model for 2021. Children 2021;8(2):139.
53. Robinson C, Gund A, Sjoqvist BA, et al. Using telemedicine in the care of newborn infants after discharge from a neonatal intensive care unit reduced the need of hospital visits. Acta Paedatr 2016;105(8):902–9.
54. DeMauro SB, Duncan AF, Hurt H. Telemedicine use in neonatal follow-up programs—What can we do and what we can't—Lessons learned from COVID-19. Sem Perinatol 2021;45(5):151430.
55. Saad M, Chan S, Nguyen L, et al. Patient perceptions of the benefits and barriers of virtual postnatal care: a qualitative study. BMC Preg Childbirth 2021;21:543.
56. Curfman A, Hackell JM, Herendeen NE, et al. Telehealth: Improving Access to and Quality of Pediatric Health Care. Pediatrics 2021;148(3):e2021053129.
57. Fiks AG, Jenssen BP, Ray KN. A Defining Moment for Pediatric Primary Care Telehealth 2021;175(1):9–10. https://doi.org/10.1001/jamapediatrics.2020.1881.
58. Janvier A, Lantos J, Aschner J, et al. Stronger and More Vulnerable: A Balanced View of the Impacts of the NICU Experience on Parents. Pediatrics 2016;138(3): e20160655. https://doi.org/10.1542/peds2016-0655.

59. Rosenbaum P, Gorter JW. The 'F-words' in childhood disability: I swear this is how we should think. Child Care Health Dev 2012;38(4):457–63.
60. Banihani R, Capone G, Church P, et al. The DS-ASD Diagnostic Evaluation Process: What to Expect. In: Froehlke M, Sattel R, editors. When down syndrome and autism intersect: a guide to DS-ASD for parents and professionals. 2nd Edition. Denver: Passion Flower Press; 2024.
61. Provincial Council for Maternal and Child Health. Neonatal Follow-Up Clinics Final Report. 2015. Available at: https://www.pcmch.on.ca/wp-content/uploads/Neonatal_Followup_Clinics_Final_Report_2015.pdf.
62. Provincial Council for Maternal and Child Health. Neonatal Follow-Up Implementation Strategy Final Report. 2017. Available at: https://www.pcmch.on.ca/wp-content/uploads/2022/02/NNFUImplementationWorkGroupFinalReport_2017NOV09.pdf.
63. Cohen E, Berry JG, Sanders L, et al. Status Complexicus? The Emergence of Pediatric Complex Care. Pediatrics 2018;141(S3):S202–11.
64. Pordes E, Gordon J, Sanders LM, et al. Models of Care Delivery for Children with Medical Complexity. Pediatrics 2018;141(S3):S212–23.
65. Treyvaud K, Spittle A, Anderson PJ, et al. A multilayered approach is needed in the NICU to support parents after the preterm birth of their child. Early Human Dev 2019;139:104838.
66. Mendelson T, Cluxton-Keller F, Vullo GC, et al. NICU-based Interventions To Reduce Maternal Depressive and Anxiety Symptoms: A Meta-analysis. Pediatrics 2017;139(3):e20161870.
67. vanDis EAM, van Veen SC, Hagenaars MA, et al. Long-term Outcomes of Cognitive Behavioral Therapy for Anxiety Related Disorders. A Systematic Review and Meta-analysis. JAMA Psychiatr 2020;77(3):265–73.
68. Orkin J, Major N, Esser K, et al. Coached, Coordinated, Enhanced Neonatal Transition (CCENT): protocol for a multicenter pragmatic randomized controlled trial of transition-to-home support for parents of high-risk infants. BMJ Open 2021;11:e046706. https://doi.org/10.1136/bmjopen-2020-046706.
69. Brazelton TB, Sparrow JD. Touchpoints. *2nd Edition*. Cambridge: Da Capo Press; 2006.
70. Synnes A, Lam MM, Ricci MF, et al. How to measure patient and family important outcomes in extremely preterm infants: a scoping review. Acta Paediatr 2024. revision pending review.
71. Kamity R, Kapavarapu PK, Chandel A. Feeding Problems and Long-Term Outcomes in Preterm Infants—A Systematic Approach to Evaluation and Management. Children 2021;8(12):1158.
72. Halfon N, Hochstein M. Life course health development: An integrated framework for developing health, policy, and research. Milbank Q 2002;80:433–79.
73. Litt JS, Halfon N, Msall ME, et al. Ensuring Optimal Outcomes for Preterm Infants after NICU Discharge: A Life Course Health Development Approach to High-Risk Infant Follow-Up. Children 2024;11:146.

Tools for Improving Access to Subspecialty Care Among Rural Children

Genevieve Whiting, MD[a,b,*], James C. Bohnhoff, MD, MS[a,b]

KEYWORDS

• Access • Rural • Pediatric • Specialty care • Telemedicine • Referral

KEY POINTS

- Children in rural areas face increased barriers to accessing pediatric specialty care.
- Multiple access tools exist to improve rural access, including televisits, electronic consultations, and tele-mentoring, most of which involve increased effort and responsibility on the part of rural primary care providers.
- Health systems and policymakers must support primary care providers in the use of access tools to improve the care of their patients.

INTRODUCTION

Children living in rural areas encounter unique, significant barriers to the receipt of health care, including pediatric specialty care. In this article, the authors review these barriers and, taking the perspective of the primary care practitioners caring for children in rural areas, evaluate the advantages and limitations of various access tools intended to better connect children to specialty care. They highlight the potential of some access tools to increase rural primary care physicians' skill and involvement in their patient care, but also the risks of increasing rural primary care providers' workload and responsibilities without increasing their resources. They contextualize these benefits and risks within the quintuple aims advanced by the Institute of Healthcare Improvement.

ACCESS TO PEDIATRIC SPECIALTY CARE AMONG CHILDREN IN RURAL AREAS

Over 13 million children in the United States live in rural areas, which are defined by smaller size settlements and low rates of commuting to nearby larger settlements.[1,2] The ability of these children to access pediatric specialty care may be impacted by

[a] MaineHealth Pediatrics, 22 Bramhall Street, Portland, ME 04102, USA; [b] Tufts University School of Medicine, 136 Harrison Avenue, Boston, MA 02111, USA
* Corresponding author. 1 Harnois Avenue, Suite 1a, Westbrook, ME 04092.
E-mail address: Genevieve.whiting@mainehealth.org

Pediatr Clin N Am 72 (2025) 111–121
https://doi.org/10.1016/j.pcl.2024.07.022 **pediatric.theclinics.com**
0031-3955/25/

their rural locations in multiple ways. Rural areas have decreased health care infrastructure, including a lack of local pediatric hospitals,[3,4] emergency care,[5] and specialists.[6] Due to limited local pediatric care, rural families may need to travel greater distances to care. Perversely, however, rurality is also associated with transportation challenges including limited public transportation.[7] Other urban–rural differences affecting health include higher rates of tobacco use and less healthy diets and higher rates of obesity.[8,9] With these increased risk factors for chronic disease, rural children would be expected to need pediatric specialty care at higher rates than their urban counterparts, but in fact they utilize specialty care less.[10]

PRIMARY CARE IN RURAL AMERICA

Children are generally directed to pediatric specialty care from their primary care medical homes, which have unique features in rural America. Pediatric patients may receive primary care from a Pediatric or Family Medicine Physician, Nurse Practitioner, or Physician's Assistant. The American Medical Association estimates that 95% of pediatricians work in areas designated as urban and only 12% of primary care physicians (Internal Medicine, Pediatrics, and Family Medicine) work in rural communities. Metropolitan counties have 5 times the number of pediatricians per 100,000 population as noncore rural counties and 5% of counties in the United States have no primary care physician.[11,12] This would suggest that rural children are more likely than their urban counterparts to have a primary care provider who is an advanced practice provider rather than a physician.

Rural practitioners have variable associations and affiliations with larger academic medical centers in or near which most specialty pediatric care resides and through which most research on access interventions is conducted. Some practitioners will have limited or no direct relationships with pediatric specialty providers. The presence or absence of direct affiliations or indirect associations may dictate how specialty care is delivered to rural pediatric patients. However, these rural primary care practitioners may have deep and significant knowledge of their patients and their community, local resources, and barriers to care.[13]

EVALUATING THE AVAILABLE TOOLS FOR IMPROVING RURAL ACCESS TO SUBSPECIALTY CARE

Although children in rural areas face disproportionate barriers in accessing specialty care, a growing kit of access tools exists to facilitate care receipt. Some of these tools were developed specifically to reduce transportation barriers among patients. Others have been developed to address local and national shortages of subspecialists by increasing a Primary Care Provider's (PCP's) capacity to deliver "specialty level" care, a shift that can represent both a challenge and opportunity to rural PCPs. Access tools also vary in their potential to improve access to specialty care among rural children and resources they require of patients, PCPs, and specialists. The best access tool for an individual patient will depend on the patient's individual needs and barriers to care, as well as the resources of the patient, their medical home, and broader medical system.[14,15] There is relatively little research comparing different access tools to each other, and more research is needed to understand the experiences of clinicians and patients in using different access tools, as well as the health outcomes of different tools. Guided by the available literature, however, we summarize the features of several access strategies later in the following paragraphs and in **Table 1**. Our general approach is to compare each access tool to a traditional subspecialist referral, focusing on the experiences of rural patients and their primary care providers.

Table 1
A rural PCPs toolkit for improving rural access to pediatric subspecialty care

Tool	Overcomes Geographic Barriers	Reduces Demand for Subspecialists	Physical Examination	Patient Requirements (Beyond Visit with PCP)	Primary Care Provider Requirements	Specialist Requirements
Traditional Referral *Patient is scheduled to see a specialist in-person*			Specialist	Travel to specialist, Visit time		Visit time
Televisit *Patient meets virtually with a specialist*	**	N	Specialist (limited)	AV device, Internet service		Visit time, AV device, software, Internet service
Teleconference *Patient, PCP, and specialist meet virtually*	*	N	PCP with specialist guidance	Travel (local), Visit time	Visit time, Coordination, AV device, software, Internet service, Coordination with specialist	Visit time, coordination, AV device, software, Internet service, Coordination with PCP
Outreach clinics *Specialist holds clinics in locations with access barriers*	*	N	Specialist	Travel (local), Visit time		Visit time, travel time
eConsult *PCP sends questions asynchronously to specialist*	**	Y	PCP		EHR linked to specialist, time	eConsult system, time

(*continued on next page*)

Table 1
(*continued*)

Tool	Overcomes Geographic Barriers	Reduces Demand for Subspecialists	Physical Examination	Patient Requirements (Beyond Visit with PCP)	Primary Care Provider Requirements	Specialist Requirements
Tele-mentoring *Specialist provides virtual, interactive guidance to PCP*	*	Y	PCP		Time for education, additional management	Time for education
Referral Guidelines *Specialist prepares asynchronous referral guidance for PCP*	*	Y	PCP		Referral pattern changes, additional management	Guideline development

Overcomes Geographic Barriers: ** requires no travel of patients, * may still require additional travel to PCP, to outreach clinic, or to specialist office if referred.

Televisits—Patient Meets Virtually with a Specialist

Because telemedicine visits allow patients to communicate directly with specialists without travel, this tool should be of disproportionate value to rural patients for whom travel to a subspecialist is particularly burdensome. However, telemedicine visits share some limitations with in-person visits: they do not improve subspecialist shortages, will incur copays, and do not directly involve primary care providers in care.

The virtual format of telemedicine visits also conveys specific limitations. Ideally, telemedicine visits include audiovisual (AV) technology for communication and examination, which may require of patients a smart device capable of such audio–visual connection and cellular or Internet access fast and reliable enough to sustain the visit. Given the cultural differences and socioeconomic depression experienced at higher rates in rural communities, smart device ownership trails that seen in suburban and urban areas.[16] Furthermore, rural communities have less reliable cellular service, with 16% of US land and 1.4 million Americans having no LTE (long-term evolution-a standard for wireless speed and capacity for mobile devices) coverage[17] and 20 to 30% of rural Americans reporting no access to broadband Internet service.[16,18] Even if patients have devices and service to facilitate telemedicine visits, data charges may result in an additional burden of care for them. Finally, specialists may feel that virtual physical examinations are insufficient and may require rural patients to travel for initial (or all) in-person visits.[15]

Additional modifications could further reduce certain barriers to televisits. Facilities such as local medical offices, public libraries, or schools may provide private spaces, technology, and service to allow patients to connect to specialists without the burdens listed earlier (though with some degree of travel burden).

Teleconferencing—Patient, PCP, and Specialist Meet Virtually

Teleconferencing brings together a patient and providers at multiple sites. It has been studied in inpatient and emergency settings, where it can allow smaller and less specialized facilities to benefit from the knowledge of specialists at larger centers.[19,20] In outpatient pediatrics, teleconferencing can bring together patients, primary care providers, and specialists, as shown in **Fig. 1**. This visit structure is unique in that primary care providers communicate directly with specialists in real time, which could allow for more collaboration and clarification than in traditional referrals. PCPs may also perform physical examination elements in real time, providing specialists with information that may not be available through telemedicine. From a patient perspective,

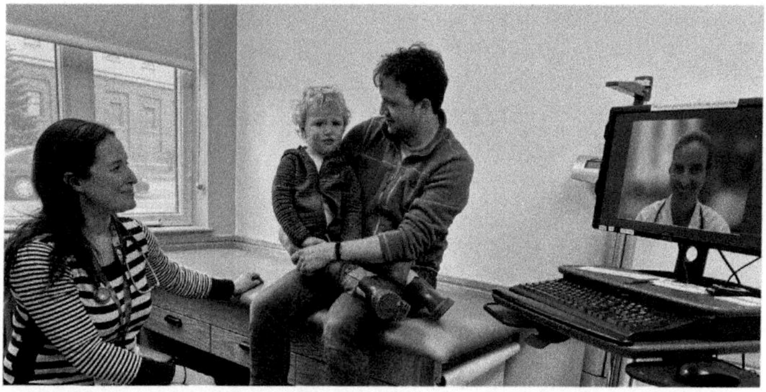

Fig. 1. In a teleconferencing visit, a primary care provider, patient, and parent virtually and synchronously connect with a specialist.

teleconferencing entails no technology or connectivity requirements and requires travel only to a (generally local) PCP office.

Teleconferencing visits are resource-intensive, requiring both PCP and specialist time, and may be limited by the difficulty of identifying a time when a patient, PCP, and specialist are all available. Perhaps for this reason, there is relatively little literature reporting implementation or outcomes associated with this access tool.

Outreach Clinics—Specialist Holds Clinics in Locations with Access Barriers

Because outreach clinics facilitate face-to-face patient-to-specialist encounters in selected rural settings, they may provide rural patients with a visit experience similar to an appointment at a clinical hub, including direct interactions with and physical examinations by specialists. However, given the disbursement of rural populations, outreach clinics may reduce travel burdens for some but remain far from others, and for no patients will transportation burdens be entirely eliminated (unlike telemedicine visits). Further, given national shortages of pediatric specialists, the lower density of patients needing specialists in rural areas, and the travel burdens outreach clinics place on specialists, outreach clinics may be scheduled infrequently enough to be inappropriate for more urgent concerns or for patients without scheduling flexibility.[21] These trade-offs for rural children and their families have not been well described. As with traditional referrals and telemedicine visits, specialist copays apply and primary care is not directly involved in the delivery of care at outreach clinics.

Electronic Consultations—PCP Sends Questions Asynchronously to Specialist

Electronic Consultations (eConsults) are an asynchronous, patient specific, provider-provider telehealth modality conducted through an electronic health records (EHR). Through eConsuls, PCPs leverage electronic health records to solicit patient-specific advice, in a timely manner (generally within several business days) without requiring a virtual or physical visit between a patient and a specialist, as illustrated in **Fig. 2**. A major aim of eConsults has been to reduce the demand for specialist care,[22,23] and for rural patients, they may also avoid many barriers inherent in traditional referrals and telemedicine visits—patients need neither travel to see a specialist, nor wait for an available subspecialty appointment. They also do not need smart devices or stable Internet or cellular connections. eConsults have the potential to increase access to care among underserved populations.[24] They also may have the secondary benefit of providing primary care providers with training that may allow them to independently manage cases they may have previously considered to require subspecialty care.[21]

eConsults have some limitations. Not all specialists or primary care providers have established systems to transmit eConsults, which generally occur through shared electronic health records. Specialist and primary care acceptance of eConsult systems will also likely depend on the ability to compensate providers for their efforts despite the lack of a visit.[25,26] Some patients prefer direct subspecialist interactions,[27] and some clinical situations (such as referrals for diagnostic tests unavailable through primary care offices) may not be appropriate for electronic consultations. Finally, eConsults add some burden to primary care providers, both through the additional information they submit in the consultation itself and in the effort of carrying out specialist recommendations.

Tele-mentoring—Specialist Provides Virtual, Interactive Guidance to PCP

If eConsults provide PCPs with patient-specific guidance first, and general guidance second, tele-mentoring flips this prioritization. The most widespread model for tele-mentoring is Project ECHO (extension for community healthcare outcomes), in which

Urology electronic consultation request:

Diagnosis: urinary incontinence

==

My clinical question is:
This patient is otherwise healthy but brings up an issue today that has been going on for "years" of post-void dribbling. She describes peeing, wiping well, then standing and when she moves she will have a "dribble." She stools daily, soft stools that can sometimes be on the runny side. Has to change her underwear frequently. Hx of anxiety. Wondering if any workup should be done or what suggestions to give to mom?

==

By indicating "Yes" below I acknowledge that consent was obtained from the patient for the performance of this eConsult. The patient understands that they may receive a bill from the subspecialty service even though they may never directly communicate with the subspecialist.
Consent obtained?: Yes

eConsult response note:

==

Clinical Question: This child's pediatrician reports that the patient has been experiencing post-void urinary dribbling. It sounds like this has been going on for over a year and can happen once or twice a day. It was reviewed at the last well-child checkup. It does not sound like there are any other concerning symptoms, including UTIs or gross hematuria. It does sound like she is otherwise fine from a urinary tract perspective. The physical exam portion of the well-child note suggests healthy and normal-appearing female external genitalia.

==

Assessment: Postvoid urinary dribbling, longstanding

==

Recommendations and contingency plan: This is a fairly benign condition, but can certainly be annoying and bothersome for the patient, especially if there is consistently wet underwear. There are a few things to double check on:
1. Constipation, even subtle and low-grade, can impinge on the bladder trigone and bladder neck, which can prevent complete emptying. We want to make sure that she is having a soft daily poop.
2. We should make sure that she is properly positioned on the toilet. Her feet should be on the ground, her legs should be spread wide enough and she should lean forward slightly, with her elbows on her knees. She should take deep breaths and make sure that she is as relaxed as possible so that her bladder can empty all the way.
3. One etiology for postvoid urinary dribbling is urinary entrapment in the vagina and vulva. If the problem persists we could double check the physical exam to make sure that there are no labial adhesions that might partially occlude urine from draining easily.

If there are no easy solutions a possible effective strategy is to "double void." She could void and then spend a brief period either wiping or even washing her hands, but sit back down to try and empty a little further in anticipation of leakage. If the problem persists despite these strategies, please let me know and I would be happy to consider further!

Fig. 2. Through electronic consultations, a PCP can solicit and receive patient-specific advice.

specialists regularly meet via audiovisual conference to discuss anonymized cases and general management principles.[28] ECHO programs are widespread and in many cases have been shown to increase provider confidence and decrease specialist referral rates.[29,30] However, tele-mentoring requires time from PCPs and mentor specialists outside of their clinical schedule. Additionally, as with eConsults, some cases are less appropriate for resolution within the primary care home, even with specialist support.

Referral Guidelines—Specialist Prepares Asynchronous Referral Guidance for PCP

Referral guidelines exist primarily to reduce rates of low acuity referrals that might be easily managed by a primary care provider in order to improve access for all patients. Referral guidelines may include such elements as appropriate PCP management before (or instead of) referral, and descriptions of situations in which referrals may be unnecessary or may be delayed.[31] Because adhering to referral guidelines shifts some decision-making and care from the specialty to primary care setting, they (like eConsults) represent one avenue for patients to receive what might be perceived as specialist-level care without traveling to specialists. However, as with eConsults, they also require additional time and effort of PCPs.

DISCUSSION

Burdens and Opportunities of Access Tools for Rural PCPs

Most access tools place some degree of burden or responsibility on PCPs. As described in **Table 1**, Teleconferences and eConsults carry technology-based requirements. Teleconferences also require PCPs to be available at times that accommodate specialists and patients. eConsults, teleconferencing, and tele-mentoring all involve an increased amount of communication and coordination between primary care and specialist sites. Finally, eConsults, tele-mentoring, and referral guidelines all aim to shift care of individual patients from specialists to primary care offices, increasing not only the volume, but the complexity of clinical care provided by PCPs. States, insurers, and health systems vary significantly in the resources and financial compensation provided for these additional efforts.[32,33]

Access tools also have potential benefits for PCPs, beyond reducing the burden of care for their patients. If care shifted into the primary care setting is reimbursed, this will ultimately financially benefit primary care offices. Providers may experience more continuity with their patients through their involvement in more specialty-level care, and providers may build their skill sets. Both patient continuity and continued education are drivers of provider satisfaction.[34,35]

Framework for Health Care Improvement—The Quintuple Aim

The Quintuple Aim is the Institute for Healthcare Improvement's framework to guide efforts to improve the US health care system by suggesting the need for harmonizing aims that otherwise might seem in conflict.[36] The 5 aims are the following:

1. Improve patient experience
2. Improve population health
3. Reduce costs
4. Reduce burnout
5. Improve equity

The challenges and opportunities inherent in efforts to improve the access to pediatric specialists for children living in rural communities align well within the framework of the quintuple aim. Access tools that avoid unnecessary travel burden aim to improve patient experiences and reduce (travel) costs. Access tools that avoid unnecessary specialist visits reduce (health care) costs. To the extent that access tools increase the number of rural patients who ultimately access subspecialty care, they support population health and equity. However, the opportunities presented for patients may pose an additional burden to the primary care system and increase burnout, unless proper resources are allocated. These include the following:

- Systems to support and compensate providers for time spent caring for higher complexity patients.
- Systems to support and compensate providers for time spent improving their skill set to deliver higher complexity care.
- Investment in electronic health records that facilitate communication with specialists.
- Resources to support primary care sites and patients in navigating their options to access specialist-level care and in utilizing high-tech care modalities.

Optimizing rural children's access to pediatric subspecialty care will require continued efforts on the part of health systems, researchers, and policymakers.

Health systems should explore ways in which they can support rural providers with the proper infrastructure and compensation models to provide their patients with specialty-level care.

Researchers should study the relative benefits of the different access tools available as well as the implementation of these tools in rural settings.

Policymakers should support measures that reimburse providers for care that occurs outside of traditional visits, such as the use of access tools.

If these efforts succeed, the effect on rural health care could be significant. Improved equity in patient access to specialist-level care could decrease urban–rural disparities in health outcomes. In addition, appropriate supports for rural PCPs may decrease their attrition and facilitate their recruitment. The shift of more (reimbursed) care from academic centers to rural primary care practices could also support the employment of additional support staff, representing a financial benefit to rural communities at large.

SUMMARY

Rural primary care physicians may have multiple options when seeking to obtain specialist-level care for their patients. These tools vary in their capacity to overcome different access barriers and in their requirements of PCPs, patients, and specialists. Because most access tools impose additional burdens on primary care providers, health care systems and policymakers should explore ways to support these efforts. Additionally, more work is needed to understand the current use of different access tools, their health outcomes, and their acceptability to patients, referrers, and specialists.

CLINICS CARE POINTS

- When a patient requires specialist-level care, consider
  - Patient-specific barriers and resources.
  - The necessity for a face-to-face specialist visit.
  - Patient preferences.
  - Available access tools.

DISCLOSURES

J.C. Bohnhoff receives support from the National Institutes of Health, United States [1K12TR004384].

REFERENCES

1. Hart LG, Larson EH, Lishner DM. Rural definitions for health policy and research. Am J Public Health 2005;95(7):1149–55.
2. Our rural communities [internet]. United States Census Bureau; 2022 [cited 2024 Feb 15]. (Census Spotlights). Available at: https://www.census.gov/library/spotlights/2020/rural.html.
3. Brown L, França UL, McManus ML. Neighborhood Poverty and Distance to Pediatric Hospital Care. Acad Pediatr 2023;23(6):1276–81.
4. Cushing AM, Bucholz EM, Chien AT, et al. Availability of Pediatric Inpatient Services in the United States. Pediatrics 2021;148(1). Available at: https://www.ncbi.nlm.nih.gov/pubmed/34127553.
5. Cushing AM, Bucholz E, Michelson KA. Trends in Regionalization of Emergency Care for Common Pediatric Conditions. Pediatrics 2020;145(4). e20192989.
6. Leslie LK, Orr CJ, Turner AL, et al. Child Health and the US Pediatric Subspecialty Workforce: Planning for the Future. Pediatrics 2024 1;153(Suppl 2). e2023063678B.
7. The U.S. Rural Population and Scheduled Intercity Transportation in 2010: A Five-Year Decline in Transportation Access. Bureau of Transportation Statistics 2011.

Available at: https://www.bts.gov/sites/bts.dot.gov/files/legacy/publications/scheduled_intercity_transportation_and_the_us_rural_population/2010/pdf/entire.pdf. [Accessed 26 January 2024].
8. Lawrence E, Hummer RA, Harris KM. The Cardiovascular Health of Young Adults: Disparities along the Urban-Rural Continuum. Ann Am Acad Pol Soc Sci 2017;672(1):257–81.
9. Crouch E, Abshire DA, Wirth MD, et al. Rural-Urban Differences in Overweight and Obesity, Physical Activity, and Food Security Among Children and Adolescents. Prev Chronic Dis 2023;20:E92.
10. Ming DY, Jones KA, White MJ, et al. Healthcare Utilization for Medicaid-Insured Children with Medical Complexity: Differences by Sociodemographic Characteristics. Matern Child Health J 2022;26(12):2407–18.
11. Supply and distribution of the primary care workforce in rural America: 2019. WWAMI Rural Health Research Center; 2020. Report No.: 167. Available at: https://depts.washington.edu/fammed/rhrc/wp-content/uploads/sites/4/2020/06/RHRC_PB167_Larson.pdf. [Accessed 1 March 2024].
12. Ramesh T, Yu H. US Pediatric Primary Care Physician Workforce in Rural Areas, 2010 to 2020. JAMA Netw Open 2023;6(9):e2333467.
13. Arora S, Kalishman S, Dion D, et al. Partnering urban academic medical centers and rural primary care clinicians to provide complex chronic disease care. Health Aff (Millwood) 2011;30(6):1176–84.
14. Bohnhoff JC, Guyon-Harris K, Schweiberger K, et al. General and subspecialist pediatrician perspectives on barriers and strategies for referral: a latent profile analysis. BMC Pediatr 2023;23(1):576.
15. Ray KN, Kahn JM. Connected Subspecialty Care: Applying Telehealth Strategies to Specific Referral Barriers. Acad Pediatr 2020;20(1):16–22, 2019/08/14 ed.
16. Vogels Emily. Some digital divides persist between rural, urban and suburban America [Internet]. Pew Research Center; 2021. Available at: https://www.pewresearch.org/short-reads/2021/08/19/some-digital-divides-persist-between-rural-urban-and-suburban-america/. [Accessed 15 February 2024].
17. Wheeler T. Improving wireless coverage in rural America [internet]. FCC Blog; 2016. Available at: https://www.fcc.gov/news-events/blog/2016/10/27/improving-wireless-coverage-rural-america. [Accessed 15 February 2024].
18. 2020 Broadband Deployment Report [Internet]. Federal Communications Commission. 2020. Report No.: FCC 20-50. Available at: https://docs.fcc.gov/public/attachments/FCC-20-50A1.pdf. [Accessed 15 February 2024].
19. Kim EW, Teague-Ross TJ, Greenfield WW, et al. Telemedicine collaboration improves perinatal regionalization and lowers statewide infant mortality. J Perinatol 2013;33(9):725–30.
20. Brova M, Boggs KM, Zachrison KS, et al. Pediatric Telemedicine Use in United States Emergency Departments. Acad Emerg Med 2018;25(12):1427–32.
21. Gruen R, Weeramanthri T, Knight S, et al. Specialist outreach clinics in primary care and rural hospital settings (Cochrane Review). Community Eye Health 2006;19(58):31, 2007/05/12 ed.
22. Johnston DL, Murto K, Kurzawa J, et al. Use of Electronic Consultation System to Improve Access to Care in Pediatric Hematology/Oncology. J Pediatr Hematol Oncol 2017;39(7):e367–9, 2017/04/25 ed.
23. Porto A, Rubin K, Wagner K, et al. Impact of Pediatric Electronic Consultations in a Federally Qualified Health Center. Telemedicine and e-Health 2021;27(12):1379–84.

24. Naka F, Lu J, Porto A, et al. Impact of dermatology eConsults on access to care and skin cancer screening in underserved populations: A model for teledermatology services in community health centers. J Am Acad Dermatol 2018;78(2): 293–302, 2017/10/25 ed.
25. Venkatesh RD, Campbell EJ, Thiim M, et al. e-Consults in gastroenterology: An opportunity for innovative care. J Telemed Telecare 2019;25(8):499–505, 2018/07/06 ed.
26. Vimalananda VG, Dvorin K, Fincke BG, et al. Patient, Primary Care Provider, and Specialist Perspectives on Specialty Care Coordination in an Integrated Health Care System. J Ambul Care Manage 2018;41(1):15–24.
27. Ackerman SL, Gleason N, Shipman SA. Comparing Patients' Experiences with Electronic and Traditional Consultation: Results from a Multisite Survey. J Gen Intern Med 2020;35(4):1135–42.
28. Project Echo [Internet]. Available at: https://projectecho.unm.edu/. [Accessed 15 February 2024].
29. Harrison JN, Steinberg J, Wilms Floet AML, et al. Addressing Pediatric Developmental and Mental Health in Primary Care Using Tele-Education. Clin Pediatr (Phila) 2022;61(1):46–55.
30. Sun H, Green B, Zaenglein A, et al. Efficacy of pediatric dermatology Extension for Community Healthcare Outcomes (ECHO) sessions on augmenting primary care providers' confidence and abilities. Pediatr Dermatol 2022;39(3):385–8.
31. Cornell E, Chandhok L, Rubin K. Implementation of referral guidelines at the interface between pediatric primary and subspecialty care. Healthc (Amst) 2015;3(2): 74–9, 2015/07/17 ed.
32. Liddy C, Deri Armstrong C, McKellips F, et al. Choosing a Model for eConsult Specialist Remuneration: Factors to Consider. Informatics 2016;3(2).
33. RE. Coverage and Payment of Interprofessional Consultation in Medicaid and the Children's Health Insurance Program (CHIP) [Internet]. Department of Health and Human Services Centers for Medicare & Medicaid Services. 2023. Available at: https://www.medicaid.gov/sites/default/files/2023-12/sho23001.pdf. [Accessed 1 March 2024].
34. Blankfield RP, Kelly RB, Alemagno SA, et al. Continuity of care in a family practice residency program. Impact on physician satisfaction. J Fam Pract 1990;31(1): 69–73, 1990/07/01 ed.
35. Rao S, Ferris TG, Hidrue MK, et al. Physician Burnout, Engagement and Career Satisfaction in a Large Academic Medical Practice. Clin Med Res 2020; 18(1):3–10.
36. Nundy S, Cooper LA, Mate KS. The Quintuple Aim for Health Care Improvement: A New Imperative to Advance Health Equity. JAMA 2022;327(6):521–2.

Pediatric Telemedicine Consults to Improve Access to Intensive Care in Rural Environments

Rachel A. Umoren, MBBCh, MS[a,b,*], Krista Birnie, MD[b]

KEYWORDS

• Telemedicine • Telehealth • Pediatric • Neonatal • Consult • Rural • Technology • Virtual

KEY POINTS

- Recent advances in telehealth adoption have demonstrated the potential for improved outcomes through implementing pediatric telehealth in rural and remote settings.
- Pediatric telemedicine consults can be used in a variety of intensive care unit (ICU) scenarios including procedural support, resuscitation, specialty consults, and transport.
- Telemedicine consults for ICU care in rural environments improve access, cost-effectiveness, and family-centeredness.
- Challenges to adopting pediatric telemedicine consults for ICU level care include issues around training, technology, resource allocation, and attention to how implementation approaches exacerbate or improve health disparities.

INTRODUCTION

The infant mortality rate (IMR), or the death of a child before their first birthday, is 6.0 per 1000 live births in the United States and the under 5 years child mortality rate is 22.7 per 100,000 population. These statistics are high when the United States is compared with other resource-rich countries.[1] Mortality rates increase as urbanization levels decrease, with disparities in IMR increasing from 5.44 deaths per 1,000 births in large urban counties to 6.55 in rural counties.[2] The regionalization of pediatric care improves the quality of care and reduces mortality rates,[3,4] but given the distribution of pediatric specialists which favors urban areas and lack of transportation (**Fig. 1**), many pediatric patients present to smaller volume rural facilities with emergent conditions

[a] Department of Pediatrics, University of Washington, 1959 NE Pacific Street, Box 356320, Seattle, WA 98195, USA; [b] Department of Pediatrics, Seattle Children's Hospital, 4800 Sand Point Way NE, Seattle, WA 98105, USA
* Corresponding author.
E-mail address: rumoren@uw.edu

Pediatr Clin N Am 72 (2025) 123–132
https://doi.org/10.1016/j.pcl.2024.07.028 **pediatric.theclinics.com**

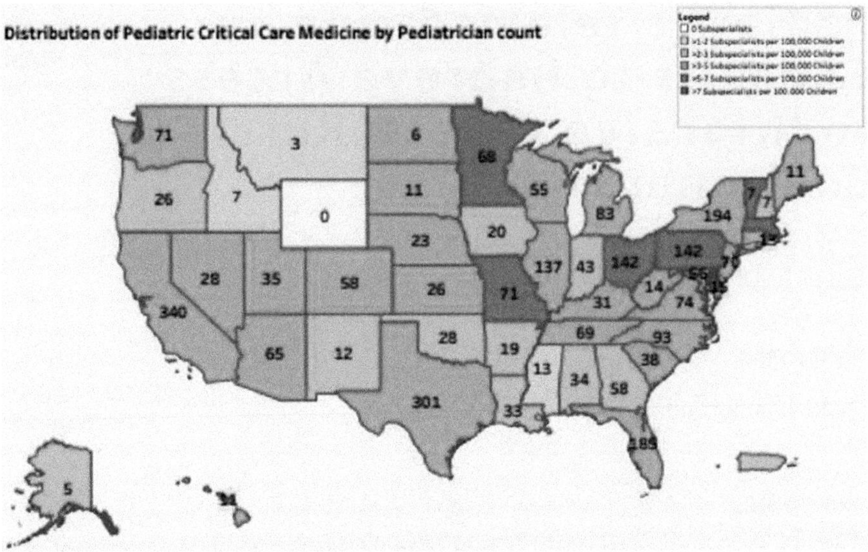

Fig. 1. Distribution of pediatric critical care medicine by pediatrician count. (Source: Pediatric Subspecialty U.S. State and County Maps | The American Board of Pediatrics (abp.org). https://www.abp.org/dashboards/pediatric-subspecialty-us-state-and-county-maps.)

requiring specialist care and are transferred to larger urban centers. When they return home, limits in public transportation may make specialist follow up challenging[5] prompting further local emergency room visits and referrals, perpetuating the cycle. Recent advances in telehealth adoption prompted by the COVID-19 pandemic have demonstrated the potential for improved outcomes through implementing pediatric telehealth in rural and remote settings.[6]

RURAL PEDIATRIC CARE AND RELEVANCE OF TELEMEDICINE

Telemedicine can improve access and quality of care for pediatric patients in underserved rural communities, reducing health care disparities and increasing provider, patient, and family satisfaction.[7] Specifically, telehealth in rural and remote emergency departments can improve clinical effectiveness, care processes, and speed of care, depending on the context and acuity of patient presentation.[8–10] While telehealth in pediatric primary care has been generally underutilized until recent years,[11,12] a range of pediatric specialist telehealth services including specialist consults in behavioral health, diabetes care[13] and obesity management, physical therapy and rehabilitation services, sleep medicine services,[14] and palliative care counseling[15] have been described.

TYPES OF TELEMEDICINE

Telemedicine can generally be classified into synchronous[16] and asynchronous or store-and-forward models.[17] Synchronous models involve using an audio and video connection to communicate in real-time and are particularly useful in acute and emergent conditions or for patients requiring intensive care. The use of synchronous telemedicine results in improved quality of care and resulted in a decrease in the transfer rate (31%–87.5%; 4 studies), a shorter length of stay (8.2 vs 15.1 d) (6 studies), a change or reinforcement of the medical care plan, a reduction in complications and illness severity, and a low hospital and standardized mortality rate.[16]

Another approach to describing telemedicine is audio-only versus video telemedicine. Audio-only or phone telemedicine is particularly useful in settings where broadband Internet availability is low and depending on the condition, patient outcomes may be generally comparable with video telemedicine.[8,18] However, in other studies, video telemedicine had added benefits in improving provider diagnostic accuracy and reducing readmission rates.[16] Video telemedicine can be provided using videoconferencing platforms with specially designed features to support telehealth such as pan-tilt-zoom cameras and the ability to use peripheral devices such as stethoscopes to remotely auscultate heart and lung sounds. These features are particularly useful for critical care and inpatient settings. However, in many ambulatory settings including home telehealth, regular video conferencing platforms may provide adequate audiovisual connection, particularly when accompanied by images sent through a Health Insurance Portability and Accountability Act (HIPAA) compliant platforms.

APPLICATIONS OF TELEHEALTH

Teleconsult

There are many examples of improved access, decreased costs, and effectively delivered care with the use of teleconsults in rural areas. Pediatric critical care teleconsults to community hospitalists is feasible and results in reduced Pediatric Intensive Care Unit (PICU) admissions.[19] Emergency rooms without pediatric emergency medicine providers have benefited from teleconsults with Pediatric Emergency Medicine (PEM) staffed Emergency Departments (EDs) and/or pediatric intensivists. These teleconsults during the initial presentation in a rural ED support the goal of managing children in their local hospitals and minimizing preventable inter-facility transfers. They have also been shown to improve management and reduce medication errors.[20] Home-based telehealth for children with medical complexity has been shown to be feasible, well received by caregivers, and may result in decreased hospitalizations.[21] Another example involves nurse-facilitated diabetes care management at remote clinics while the pediatric clinician consults via telehealth. Caregiver assessment scales reported improvements in access to care (81%), confidence in communication quality and privacy (91%), and the vast majority (98%) showed interest in the use telemedicine for future health needs.[13] Telepsychiatry is a specific example of teleconsults that have been used effectively to address mental health crises in EDs. Telepsychiatry was shown to be cost-efficient, improve clinical and operational efficiency, and improve the patient and family experience, without an increase in safety concerns based on 72 hour readmission rates.[22]

Teleresuscitation

Teleresuscitation can be used to support clinicians during high-risk newborn resuscitations with improved access to neonatology expertise. This telehealth support improves the quality of care and reduces unnecessary transfers.[23] Emergency rooms also benefit from teleresuscitation with the telehealth support of intensivist or pediatric emergency medicine expertise.[20]

Telerounding

Telerounding harnesses the use of telehealth platforms to include remote participants in daily bedside rounds. Telerounding increases family participation when parents and caregivers face barriers to being present on rounds. Many ICUs have moved toward family-centered rounding and parents place a high value on these daily encounters with their team of clinicians; however, barriers including transportation difficulties and home-to-hospital distance often make their daily in-person presence unattainable. Offering video and/or audio-only-based remote participation of parents has been shown to increase parental engagement, reduce parental stress, potentially decrease length of stay by earlier parental involvement in discharge planning, and allow for cost-savings for parents who otherwise may have lost wages or benefits if they were to be in-person for rounds everyday.[24] Telerounding also provides opportunities for specialty consultants to contribute during rounds while the entire bedside team and family is present and supports intensive care when patients are in isolation.[25]

Teleprocedure

Telehealth can be used to remotely facilitate procedures or perioperative care. In pediatric orthopedic medicine, one study compared efficacy, duration, and parental satisfaction of in-person versus telehealth visits for a 4 week postop cast removal in the setting of type I supracondylar humeral fractures or occult elbow injuries. Telehealth visits were more efficient and there were higher satisfaction scores. There was no significant difference in fracture displacement, range of motion, or pain scores between groups at the 8 week postop visit that was in person for both groups.[26] Telehealth has been studied for preoperative evaluations by pediatric hospitalists of medically complex patients undergoing elective orthopedic procedures. There was no statistically significant difference for the median number of hospitalist recommendations or progression to surgery between the in-person or telehealth consults.[27]

Teletransport

Telehealth used during transport supports facilitation advanced care prior to arrival at the receiving hospital which can lead to earlier intervention and even improved outcomes as based on recommendations from the pediatric clinicians at the receiving hospital.[20]

Teletherapy

Telehealth interventions in pediatric speech therapy and occupational therapy, though not widely used, have been shown to be successful. Teletherapy treatment has high family participation and satisfaction, as well as being clinically and cost-effective.[28]

Transitions of Care

Poor transitions of care result in increased hospital admissions and readmissions, escalation of care once hospitalized, and poor patient experience and outcomes. Telehealth can facilitate improved care by creating a supported collaboration during various transitions of care. For instance, telehealth has been shown to improve hand-offs between neonatologists and primary care providers for medically complex infants.[29] A specific outpatient example is one of nurse-practitioner-led telehealth being used to improve outpatient pediatric tracheostomy management.[30]

DISCUSSION

Benefits of Telemedicine to Rural Areas

There are countless benefits of telemedicine to rural areas. Telehealth offers opportunities to increase accessibility, cost-effectiveness, and family centeredness.[31] In one systemic review comparing satisfaction among caregivers and pediatric providers for telehealth versus in-person visits, telehealth services received more favorable or comparable satisfaction rating than in-person visits. The benefits included the "ease of use" and "reduced need for transportation." The main improvement areas related to technological challenges, a limited personal interaction with the provider, and a lack of physical examination.[32] The reduced travel time is significant in telehealth visits used for rural areas and leads to improved satisfaction in caregivers.[33] Various specialties from neonatology to palliative care have effectively employed telehealth, offering a variety of visit types.[15,34] In surgical fields, comparable services of initial consultations, preoperative visits, postoperative visits, and follow-up visits have been documented.[33]

There is evidence that telemedicine can improve the triaging of patients in emergency rooms, with early intervention from ICU specialists leading to children to arriving to receiving hospitals with lower illness severity at admission to the PICU.[35] Importantly, early telehealth intervention with corresponding protocols and communication pathways have been shown to reduce preventable transfers and keep patients closer to home.[10]

Telehealth can also decrease no-show rates because caregivers and patients have fewer barriers in getting to an in-person appointment. Decreasing no-show rates is important to improve health outcomes and decrease the overall cost burden to the health care system. In one such study of a pediatric asthma clinic, caregivers were offered the option of telehealth versus in-person follow-up visits. The no-show rate significantly decreased, and parents reported improved access, time saved, and simplicity in use.[36]

Challenges

There are many challenges to the delivery of telehealth consults to improve intensive care unit (ICU) level care in rural communities. Common challenges include issues around necessary training, accessibility, available technology, cost, resource allocation, and attention to how implementation exacerbates or improves health disparities.[37,38]

Cost

The primary barriers to telehealth, as reported in an analysis of a national representative survey of American Academy of Pediatrics post-residency member pediatricians in 2016, were insufficient payment and inability to bill for services. The study also considered what factors may convince nonusers to consider adopting telehealth. They found that 40% of nonusers would consider using telehealth for follow-up care if services significantly decreased patient travel time and improved access to specialists or pediatricians.[39] When considering issues of cost, one must consider the cost of the technology itself as well as the human resources, as well as the actual billable services and cost to the family.

Equity/Disparities

Expanding telehealth in pediatrics requires user-friendly digital health, facilitating patient preferred language, and simplifying logistical processes to avoid worsening health disparities. One study examined telemedicine use within a large pediatric primary care network and identified that use differed based on child age, race, and ethnicity, and recent preventive care, highlighting the need for further work to increase equitable access to primary care telemedicine.[40] Disparities have resulted in many medically under resourced communities, including people of color, language of care other than English, rural populations, and youth with special health care needs with additional barriers in accessing telehealth services. Disparities in access to hardware and Internet limit implementation and adoption of new technologies. Differences in digital literacy can also further worsen inequity.[41] Employing user-friendly technology, facilitating care in the patient preferred language, and simplifying logistical processes are factors that will contribute to reducing health disparities.[42]

Infrastructure

Rural telehealth infrastructure has been a major focus of funding for over two decades. Early demonstration projects supported by rural telehealth grants have formed the framework of today's telehealth infrastructure.[6] With the COVID-19 pandemic, more attention has been given to the need for infrastructure to support telehealth. While Internet connectivity is improving, broadband connections remain limited in rural settings which hinders the adoption of telehealth by rural communities.

Education/Awareness

The COVID-19 pandemic increased awareness of individuals and institutions of the benefits of telehealth. During the public health emergency, many new use cases involving inpatient and ambulatory telehealth, including "hospital at home" were explored. The success of many of these pilots has led to greater adoption of telehealth post-pandemic with most institutions continuing to maintain some telehealth appointments at a higher rate than pre-pandemic even while transitioning back to an in-person format for the majority of visits. As evidenced by a Google Scholar search, there is variable awareness and research being done on the various telehealth applications, with teleconsults and teletherapy leading the way (**Fig. 2**).

Reimbursement

Historically, telehealth visits had not been reimbursed at the same rates as in person visits.[43] However, in recent years, the institution of parity for reimbursement of telehealth visits by public and private insurers has been a major factor in increasing telehealth adoption.

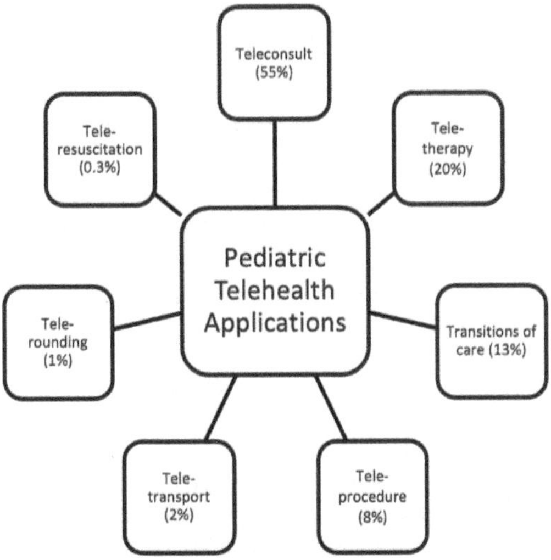

Fig. 2. Relative frequency of reported pediatric telehealth applications (n = 10,534). Google Scholar search performed on February 15, 2024 for publications from 2019 to 2023 on "pediatrics" and "<telehealth application>"

SUMMARY

With increasing centralization of care in urban centers and decreasing access to pediatric ICU specialists in remote areas, the implementation of telehealth to improve outcomes in rural ICU pediatric care is paramount. Advances in telehealth adoption have demonstrated the potential for improved pediatric ICU outcomes through implementing pediatric telehealth in rural and remote settings. Telemedicine consults can be used in a variety of ICU scenarios including procedural support, resuscitation, specialty consults, and transport. Applying the variety of uses of telemedicine in rural environments has improved access, cost-effectiveness, and family-centeredness of care. Challenges include issues around training, technology, and resource allocation. As centers introduce new technologies and increasingly use telehealth to support ICU level care, it is important to draw attention to how implementation addresses the needs of rural patients and limits health disparities.

CLINICS CARE POINTS

- Recent advances in telehealth adoption prompted by the COVID-19 pandemic have demonstrated the potential for improved outcomes through implementing pediatric telehealth in rural and remote settings.
- There are many applications of telemedicine to improve access to ICU level care in remote settings, including but not limited to teleconsult, teleresuscitation, telerounding, teletransport, and teleprocedure.
- Benefits to adopting telemedicine consults include accessibility, cost-effectiveness, and family centeredness.
- Challenges to adopting telemedicine consults include issues around necessary training, accessibility, available technology, cost, resource allocation, and attention to how implementation exacerbates or improves health disparities.

DISCLOSURE

The authors have no conflicts of interest to disclose. Dr R.A. Umoren is supported by funding from the Agency for Healthcare Research and Quality, United States (AHRQ) R18HS029607 and the Eunice Kennedy Shriver National Institute of Child Health and Human Development R01HD112327, United States.

REFERENCES

1. Chen A, Oster E, Williams H. Why is infant mortality higher in the United States than in Europe? Am Econ J Econ Pol 2016;8(2):89–124.
2. Ely DM, Driscoll AK, Matthews T. Infant mortality rates in rural and urban areas in the United States, 2014, vol 285. US Department of Health and Human Services, Centers for Disease Control; 2017.
3. Pollack MM, Alexander SR, Clarke N, et al. Improved outcomes from tertiary center pediatric intensive care: a statewide comparison of tertiary and nontertiary care facilities. Crit Care Med 1991;19(2):150–9.
4. Phibbs CS, Baker LC, Caughey AB, et al. Level and volume of neonatal intensive care and mortality in very-low-birth-weight infants. N Engl J Med 2007;356(21): 2165–75.

5. Riley T, Umoren R, Kotler A, et al. Disparities in access to healthcare services in a regional neonatal transport network. Int J Ind Ergon 2024;99:103526.
6. Patel PD, Cobb J, Wright D, et al. Rapid development of telehealth capabilities within pediatric patient portal infrastructure for COVID-19 care: barriers, solutions, results. J Am Med Inf Assoc 2020;27(7):1116–20.
7. Marcin JP, Shaikh U, Steinhorn RH. Addressing health disparities in rural communities using telehealth. Pediatr Res 2016;79(1):169–76.
8. Tsou C, Robinson S, Boyd J, et al. Effectiveness of telehealth in rural and remote emergency departments: systematic review. J Med Internet Res 2021;23(11): e30632.
9. du Toit M, Malau-Aduli B, Vangaveti V, et al. Use of telehealth in the management of non-critical emergencies in rural or remote emergency departments: a systematic review. J Telemed Telecare 2019;25(1):3–16.
10. Taylor MA, Knochel ML, Proctor SJ, et al. Pediatric trauma telemedicine in a rural state: Lessons learned from a 1-year experience. J Pediatr Surg 2021;56(2): 385–9.
11. Wenderlich AM, Herendeen N. Telehealth in pediatric primary care. Curr Probl Pediatr Adolesc Health Care 2021;51(1):100951.
12. Olson CA, McSwain SD, Curfman AL, et al. The current pediatric telehealth landscape. Pediatrics 2018;141(3). e20172334.
13. Stallings DE, Duetsch JR, Gustin TS, et al. An interdisciplinary telemedicine innovation to enhance pediatric diabetes care in rural communities: A proposed practice initiative. J Spec Pediatr Nurs (JSPN) 2023;28(2):e12405.
14. Witmans MB, Dick B, Good J, et al. Delivery of pediatric sleep services via telehealth: the Alberta experience and lessons learned. Behav Sleep Med 2008;6(4): 207–19.
15. Winegard B, Miller EG, Slamon NB. Use of Telehealth in Pediatric Palliative Care. Telemed J e Health 2017;23(11):938–40.
16. Nadar M, Jouvet P, Tucci M, et al. Impact of synchronous telemedicine models on clinical outcomes in pediatric acute care settings: a systematic review. Pediatr Crit Care Med 2018;19(12):e662–71.
17. Chan DS, Callahan CW, Sheets SJ, et al. An Internet-based store-and-forward video home telehealth system for improving asthma outcomes in children. Am J Health Syst Pharm 2003;60(19):1976–81.
18. Rush KL, Howlett L, Munro A, et al. Videoconference compared to telephone in healthcare delivery: a systematic review. Int J Med Inf 2018;118:44–53.
19. Harvey JB, Yeager BE, Cramer C, et al. The Impact of Telemedicine on Pediatric Critical Care Triage. Pediatr Crit Care Med 2017;18(11). https://doi.org/10.1097/PCC.0000000000001330.
20. Schinasi DA, Atabaki SM, Lo MD, et al. Telehealth in pediatric emergency medicine. Curr Probl Pediatr Adolesc Health Care 2021;51(1). https://doi.org/10.1016/j.cppeds.2021.100953.
21. Gentile EM, Notario PM, Amidon M, et al. Using Telehealth to Care for Children with Medical Complexity. J Pediatr Health Care 2019;33(4). https://doi.org/10.1016/j.pedhc.2019.04.005.
22. Thomas JF, Novins DK, Hosokawa PW, et al. The use of telepsychiatry to provide cost-efficient care during pediatric mental health emergencies. Psychiatr Serv 2018;69(2). https://doi.org/10.1176/appi.ps.201700140.
23. Fang JL, Chuo J. Using telehealth to support pediatricians in newborn care. Curr Probl Pediatr Adolesc Health Care 2021;51(1). https://doi.org/10.1016/j.cppeds.2021.100952.

24. Yager PH. Remote Parent Participation in Intensive Care Unit Rounds. Pediatr Clin 2020;67(4). https://doi.org/10.1016/j.pcl.2020.04.008.
25. Umoren RA, Gray MM, Handley S, et al. In-hospital telehealth supports care for neonatal patients in strict isolation. Am J Perinatol 2020;37(08):857–60.
26. Silva M, Delfosse EM, Aceves-Martin B, et al. Telehealth: A novel approach for the treatment of nondisplaced pediatric elbow fractures. J Pediatr Orthop Part B 2019;28(6). https://doi.org/10.1097/BPB.0000000000000576.
27. Goldner H, Barfchin S, Fingado EK, et al. Preoperative hospitalist telehealth visits for medically complex children during the COVID-19 pandemic. Hosp Pediatr 2022;12(12). https://doi.org/10.1542/hpeds.2021-006184.
28. Fishman GD, Elkins J. Covid-19 lessons from the field: toward a pediatric physical therapy telehealth framework. Int J Telerehabilitation 2022;14(1). https://doi.org/10.5195/ijt.2022.6448.
29. Hoffman K, Olson C, Zenge J, et al. The use of telehealth to improve handoffs between neonatologists and primary care providers for medically complex infants. Telemedicine and e-Health 2023;29(10). https://doi.org/10.1089/tmj.2022.0400.
30. Moreno L, Peck JL. Nurse Practitioner–Led Telehealth to Improve Outpatient Pediatric Tracheostomy Management in South Texas. J Pediatr Health Care 2020; 34(3). https://doi.org/10.1016/j.pedhc.2019.11.008.
31. Camden C, Silva M. Pediatric teleheath: Opportunities created by the COVID-19 and suggestions to sustain its use to support families of children with disabilities. Phys Occup Ther Pediatr 2021;41(1):1–17.
32. Kodjebacheva GD, Culinski T, Kawser B, et al. Satisfaction with telehealth services compared with nontelehealth services among pediatric patients and their caregivers: systematic review of the literature. JMIR Pediatrics and Parenting 2023;6. https://doi.org/10.2196/41554.
33. Kim EN, Tyrell R, Moss WD, et al. Implementation of Telehealth in a Pediatric Plastic Surgery Clinic: A Single Center's Response to COVID-19. Ann Plast Surg 2022; 88(6):589–93.
34. Lapcharoensap W, Lund K, Huynh T. Telemedicine in neonatal medicine and resuscitation. Curr Opin Pediatr 2021;33(2):203–8.
35. Dayal P, Hojman NM, Kissee JL, et al. Impact of telemedicine on severity of illness and outcomes among children transferred from referring emergency departments to a children's hospital PICU. Pediatr Crit Care Med 2016;17(6). https://doi.org/10.1097/PCC.0000000000000761.
36. Van Houten L, Deegan K, Siemer M, et al. A telehealth initiative to decrease no-show rates in a pediatric asthma mobile clinic. J Pediatr Nurs 2021;59:143–50.
37. Brophy PD. Overview on the Challenges and Benefits of Using Telehealth Tools in a Pediatric Population. Adv Chron Kidney Dis 2017;24(1). https://doi.org/10.1053/j.ackd.2016.12.003.
38. Utidjian L, Abramson E. Pediatric telehealth: opportunities and challenges. Pediatric Clinics 2016;63(2):367–78.
39. Sisk B, Alexander J, Bodnar C, et al. Pediatrician attitudes toward and experiences with telehealth use: results from a national survey. Academic pediatrics 2020;20(5):628–35.
40. Schweiberger K, Hoberman A, Iagnemma J, et al. Practice-level variation in telemedicine use in a pediatric primary care network during the COVID-19 pandemic: retrospective analysis and survey study. J Med Internet Res 2020; 22(12):e24345.

41. Curfman A, Hackell JM, Herendeen NE, et al. Telehealth: Opportunities to Improve Access, Quality, and Cost in Pediatric Care. Pediatrics 2022;149(3). e2021056035.
42. Jones SA, Sara, Yared A, et al. Direct-to-Patient Telehealth Equity: Reaching Diverse Pediatric Populations in Primary Care. Fam Syst Health 2022;41(1):61–7.
43. Wade VA, Karnon J, Elshaug AG, et al. A systematic review of economic analyses of telehealth services using real time video communication. BMC Health Serv Res 2010;10:233.

Innovative Technology to Improve Simulation Access for Rural Clinicians

Allison Zanno, MD[a,b,*], Jeffrey Holmes, MD[c,d],
Michael Ferguson, MBBS, MTeach[a,e], Misty Melendi, MD[a,b]

KEYWORDS

• Simulation • Telesimulation • Rural clinicians • Medical education • Mixed reality
• Mobile simulation

KEY POINTS

- Access to health care simulation for rural clinicians is important for team-based training.
- There are many different types of simulation modalities to help address geographic and financial barriers to simulation in rural areas.
- Telesimulation and Augmented Reality simulation offer alternatives to traditional simulation for high-acuity, low-occurance (HALO) events.

INTRODUCTION

Ensuring access to high-quality neonatal and pediatric medical care, regardless of geographic location, is a critical component of public health with profound implications for the well-being of our youngest population. Recent data suggest that as much as 15% to 20% of the population, including 1 in 5 children,[1] live in rural areas and encounter a higher burden of health care disparities compared with their urban counterparts. As rural health care providers struggle with constrained resources, geographic isolation, and a shortage of trained professionals, the delivery of timely

[a] Department of Pediatrics, Tufts University School of Medicine, Boston, MA, USA; [b] Department of Pediatrics, Section of Neonatal–Perinatal Medicine, The Barbara Bush Children's Hospital at Maine Medical Center, 22 Bramhall Street, Coloumbe Family Tower, 4th Floor, Suite 4809, Portland, ME 04102, USA; [c] Department of Emergency Medicine, Tufts University School of Medicine, Boston, MA, USA; [d] The Hannaford Center for Safety, Innovation and Simulation, Maine Medical Center, 22 Bramhall Street, Coloumbe Family Tower, 4th Floor, Suite 4809, Portland, ME 04102, USA; [e] Department of Pediatrics, Section of Pediatric Intensive Care, The Barbara Bush Children's Hospital at Maine Medical Center, 22 Bramhall Street, Coloumbe Family Tower, 4th Floor, Suite 4809, Portland, ME 04102, USA
* Corresponding author. Barbara Bush Children's Hospital at Maine Medical Center, 22 Bramhall Street, Columbe Family Tower, 4th Floor, Suite 4809, Portland, ME 04102.
E-mail address: Allison.Zanno@mainehealth.org

Pediatr Clin N Am 72 (2025) 133–150
https://doi.org/10.1016/j.pcl.2024.07.023 **pediatric.theclinics.com**
0031-3955/25/

and effective pediatric care becomes increasingly difficult.[2] The repercussions are particularly dire for high-acuity, low-occurrence (HALO) events, such as acute resuscitation, where swift intervention can be the difference between life and death. Studies consistently highlight the disparities in health care delivery between rural and urban settings where pediatric volume and readiness for emergencies play a large role. For example, children who present to emergency departments with limited pediatric readiness have been found to have increased mortality,[3,4] and pediatric patients are twice as likely to die if they suffer a cardiac arrest in a rural hospital compared with in a specialty children's hospital.[5]

Access to structured pediatric training is critical in addressing health care disparities. Unfortunately, one of the persistent challenges in rural areas is the limited availability of specialized health care services. Almost half of all counties in the United States are without a general pediatrician, and 82% lack one in rural areas,[6] with pediatric specialists being even more scarce.[7] The American Hospital Association found that between 2008 and 2018, the number of pediatric inpatient units decreased by almost 20%, mostly affecting rural areas. These closures have led to a significant increase in distance to the nearest pediatric inpatient unit for almost one-quarter of US children.[8–10] These rural challenges highlight the need to identify innovative educational opportunities to support hospitals in rural areas with lower pediatric volumes to maintain skills and readiness and address this rural/urban disparity.

Many physicians report lower confidence and skill with procedures as time away from residency increases. Iyer and colleagues[11] showed that pediatricians reported feeling less prepared in procedural skills in practice than at graduation and would require additional training. Multiple studies have suggested that educational collaboratives between more general hospitals in rural areas and children's hospitals can support access and quality of pediatric care.[12,13] Geography is often a barrier, as distance can limit education opportunities. However, the integration of technology in medical education has the potential to bridge this geographic gap.

One notable example of technology-driven medical education is health care simulation training. Simulation training is a widely accepted deliberate practice methodology to improve skills, including technical and task-related skills, communication, and team performance. Simulation programs allow health care providers in rural areas to practice for pediatric HALO events in a low-risk environment, honing their skills and building confidence.[14,15] Simulation programs have been shown to enhance clinical performance, reduce errors, and improve overall patient outcomes. Recent evidence has shown simulation-based training significantly impacted medical professionals' competency and confidence levels, particularly in specialties like neonatology.[16] Neonatal resuscitation simulation training decreases neonatal mortality and is an ideal method to train interprofessional teams. Furthermore, consensus statements from the International Liaison Committee on Resuscitation (ILCOR) and the American Heart Association (AHA) consistently recommend frequent simulation sessions to optimize skills.[17]

Team-based training, such as those afforded by simulation and associated educational opportunities, can potentially improve hospital staff recruitment and retention.[18–21] Engagement is crucial to maintaining the workforce and helping prevent hospital closures because of a lack of staffing. Hospital staff engagement has been shown to be directly related to patient safety, whereas hospitals with increased engagement have lower adverse safety events.[22,23]

The existing disparities in pediatric infant and neonatal medical care in rural areas underscore the urgent need for innovative solutions. Integrating simulation technology in medical education and continuing medical education offers an approach to address these challenges, empowering rural health care providers with access to training opportunities to deliver high-quality care. This article reviews existing simulation modalities that play an important role in narrowing the gap between urban and rural pediatric health care outcomes. Specifically, it outlines the terminology, the application or implementation strategy of the technology, the benefits and limitations associated with the modality, and future directions.

SIMULATION TECHNOLOGIES

Mobile Simulation

Traditional health care simulation typically occurs at or near simulation centers that are affiliated with academic medical centers ("center-based simulation"). Providing access to rural care teams presents logistical challenges (ie, distance traveled to the simulation center, limited clinical coverage during training). Building additional simulation centers across rural regions is not typically financially viable owing to construction and ongoing operating costs.[24] Mobile simulation, however, is a solution to some of these challenges. It is defined as the "ability to move the simulator from one teaching location to another or teach a scenario on the move"[25] (**Fig. 1**). This transportable simulation allows simulation centers to bring training and technology to rural hospitals. Physically, this can be as a mobile simulation training unit in the form of a bus, trailer, or ambulance that replicates a clinical setting[26] or by bringing simulators to train in the hospital's actual clinical space, termed in situ simulation (ISS). The remainder of this section addresses mobile ISS simulation, including modalities, benefits, challenges, program implementation, and future directions.

Implementation of mobile simulation

ISS is defined as a simulation that takes place "in the actual patient care setting/environment in an effort to achieve a high level of fidelity or realism."[25] Different simulation modalities are used in mobile simulation training, including manikins and/or embedded simulated persons. Manikin-based simulation uses human-like manikins to create a patient encounter via heart and lung sounds, palpable pulses, voice interactions, vital signs monitoring, and limited movement. If financial resources are limited, more lower-fidelity manikins can be used effectively.[27–32] Embedded simulated persons are individuals trained to portray either patients or family members. They can be used independently or as an effective adjunct in a mixed-method ISS.

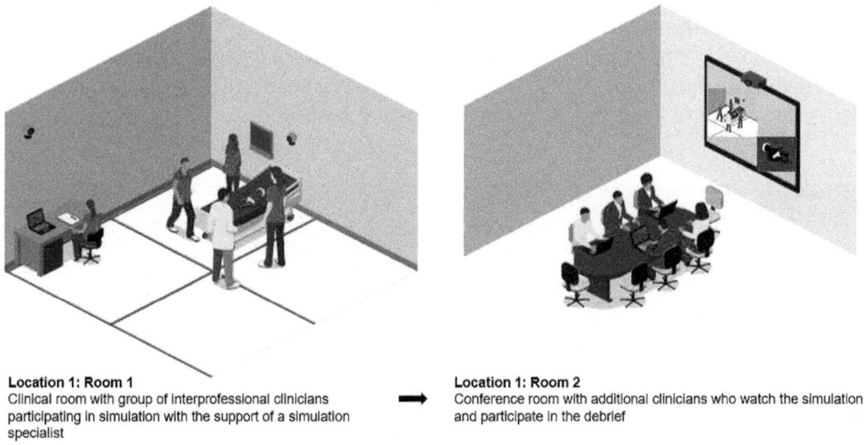

Location 1: Room 1
Clinical room with group of interprofessional clinicians participating in simulation with the support of a simulation specialist
Location 1: Room 2
Conference room with additional clinicians who watch the simulation and participate in the debrief

Fig. 1. Mobile in situ simulation setup example.

Although training teams in communication, technical skills, and teamwork is necessary for improved patient safety, single or infrequent sessions are not sufficient to maintain skill levels.[33,34] Gains in cognitive, procedural, communication, and teamwork domains decay over time without regular reinforcement or refresher training.[33,34] To maximize potential gains from ISS, education should be more explicitly connected with health service priorities and patient outcomes. This has been coined "translational simulation," a functional description of a subset of simulation activities that, in addition to training individuals and teams, is directly focused on improving health care processes and outcomes.[35] Education and training are directed at a specific health care outcome target, with the goal of service improvements and a change in patient outcomes. Designing ISS events with this forethought can allow them to be tailored to specific rural health care needs, promoting relevance and applicability.

Several ISS programs have been able to show a translational impact of their training by explicitly integrating them into quality improvement projects. Abulebda and colleagues[13] demonstrated an interventional study to measure and improve the community emergency department's Pediatric Readiness Survey (PRS) scores, a composite readiness score shown to correlate with decreased mortality in critically ill children.[3,36] This program consisted of ISS, report-outs, access to online pediatric readiness resources, and content experts, which demonstrated significant improvement in pediatric readiness scores. The improvement was attributable to tailoring scenarios to focus on components of the PRS. The simulation-based performance of real-world teams applying their knowledge, using their equipment, and accessing their guidelines provided emergency department leaders with information on gaps in the care for sick children. Their simulation program demonstrated the value of strong communication and collaboration between community hospitals and academic medical centers.

Benefits of mobile simulation

Numerous benefits are obtained by providing rural care teams access to ISS. Realistic re-enactment of clinical scenarios can provide deliberate practice opportunities to improve teamwork and communication.[37] Teamwork training is a specific recommendation by the Joint Commission, as communication issues top the list of identifiable root causes of infant death and injury during delivery and subsequent resuscitation. Although cost is often a barrier in creating large simulation centers and in high-fidelity (Hi-Fi) simulation, many task trainers and other low-cost options exist, which could be useful for ISS and mobile simulation in lower-resource settings.[38] Most importantly, interprofessional in situ allows for a postsimulation reflective practice (**Fig. 2**), termed "debriefing." Debriefing, when led by skilled simulation educators, can serve as a forum for participants to identify areas of potential improvement in teamwork, medical knowledge, and their hospital system.

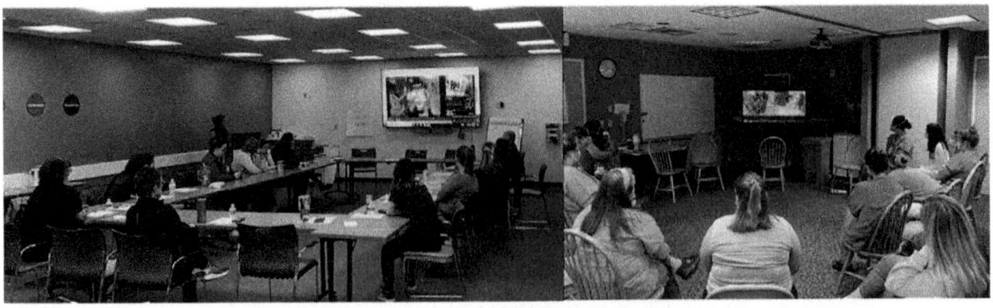

Fig. 2. ISS example of clinicians. Viewing and debriefing from a separate room.

Limitations of mobile simulation

The use of ISS in rural settings has many drawbacks, including the availability of training spaces, scheduling challenges, and the cost of supplies. By using clinical spaces at the rural site, ISS can place strain on patient care. Rural hospitals may have limited space to care for patients, resulting in a higher rate of training cancellations if potential simulation space is needed for patient care. Sessions may be difficult to schedule, given the smaller pool of providers covering active clinical duties. Multiple ISS sessions may have to be scheduled to maximize participation, increasing the need for simulation experts to travel large distances. Improved operational efficiency may be gained from teams practicing with real supplies; however, the cost of using these supplies must be budgeted. ISS requires its own diligent safety practices to ensure patient readiness of clinical spaces if the need arises. Mitigation methods must be put in place to label supplies and medication effectively, ensuring they do not accidently get used for actual patient care.[39,40] Ultimately, ISS requires flexibility, as each hospital's needs, resources, and limitations will vary (**Table 1**).

Future directions of mobile simulation

Although health care simulation shows promise as an educational modality for rural health care teams, there is a need for further research on its long-term impact on service improvements, patient outcomes, and cost-effectiveness. Given the limited financial resources of rural hospitals, strategic funding support for the integration of simulation training into rural training will be critical. Increasing repeated accessibility of simulation is another frontier that merits further exploration. Given the finite simulation resources accessible to rural teams, cheaper, faster alternatives need to be explored. Although these methods may be considered "lower technology," they can

Table 1
Advantages and challenges of using mobile simulation

Advantages	Challenges
Interprofessional realistic re-enactment of scenarios	Increased probability of participants being distracted by patient care
Participants are more comfortable in their own clinical space	Higher rate of cancellations if clinical space is needed for patient care
Participants do not have to travel to simulation centers	Strain on the simulation center to bring equipment and trained facilitators to rural hospitals
Participants practice with real supplies and equipment	Cost of practicing with real supplies
Debriefing fosters team conversation to identify areas of potential improvement in teamwork, medical knowledge, and their health system	Use of clinical spaces strains resources for actual patients
The opportunity to maximize interdisciplinary participation	Safety threat of simulation materials being accidently used for actual patient care[41]
Simulation events can more effectively integrate into a local quality improvement program	Safety threat of real clinical supplies and space being used for simulation and not adequately readied for patient care postsimulation
Hospital patients and family members may see simulation practice as confidence builder	Supportive audiovisual technology is harder to put in place

still maintain psychological fidelity, are thought to be essential for effective learning, and are associated with improved retention and long-term recall.[42–45]

Telesimulation

Telesimulation, also known as "distance simulation," provides an innovative solution to address disparities in access to simulation training for neonatal and pediatric care in rural hospitals.[46] Telesimulation pairs simulation technology with audiovisual (AV) cameras allowing rural clinicians to participate in their own local environment while expert facilitators observe and provide feedback from a remote location. This enables teams to realize the benefits of ISS (**Table 2**): improving procedural skills, clinical knowledge, teamwork, and communication and identifying systems issues and latent safety threats specific to that local environment.[46] The use of telesimulation experienced rapid expansion during the COVID-19 pandemic and can be used deliberately to practice HALO events, including neonatal and pediatric resuscitations.[47–50] This section explores the setup and implementation of telesimulation, focusing on benefits, challenges, and future directions.

Implementation of telesimulation

Telesimulation requires a simulation manikin (ranging from task trainers to Hi-Fi manikins) and telecommunication equipment (ranging in capability and cost from smartphones to AV equipment designed specifically for simulation) at the local site with an Internet connection to remotely transmit audio and video data to simulation and content experts who facilitate[48] (**Fig. 3**) the simulation. The participants remain in their hospital and their clinical space with access to the same equipment and resources accessible during real HALO events. The manikin and AV equipment are within their clinical environment, live streaming to the remote facilitators, bridging any distance and reducing the cost of training.[46] A local simulation champion can be used to operate the manikin and facilitate training onsite. The use of a remote simulation manikin controller is an alternative to having a local champion.[51,62] Communicating through the AV system, facilitators lead a debrief with participants following the simulation scenario (**Fig. 4**). Successful implementation of a telesimulation program requires commitment from the local team, the remote simulation, and experienced clinical faculty, as well as administrative support.[46] Furthermore, *Simulation in Healthcare* published the development of simulation educator guidelines for distance simulation,[65] which is critical for standardization in continuing to advance the field.[66]

Barriers to implementing telesimulation

There are numerous barriers to successfully implementing a telesimulation program in rural environments. Successful implementation requires technology infrastructure and resources, which may be a barrier in limited-resourced hospitals that cannot afford equipment and/or do not have access to high-speed Internet.[49] In addition, the equipment used in telesimulation training may be unfamiliar to rural health care teams, requiring a strong partnership with simulation and content experts to ensure the adoption, implementation, and acceptance of the training modality. Although more cost-effective than ISS and mobile simulation, telesimulation still requires investing in simulation equipment, limiting accessibility in low-resourced settings with limited financial resources. Thus, implementing telesimulation in rural hospitals not affiliated with larger health networks may be more difficult without access to financial resources to purchase equipment. Grant and philanthropic funding may be necessary to overcome this barrier at rural community hospitals that are not affiliated with academic medical centers. Although telesimulation provides valuable educational experience

Table 2
Benefits of telesimulation

Accessibility and frequency of training	• Reduces geographic barriers, improving access to simulation training for rural health care teams • Removes need for the rural team to travel to urban simulation centers for center-based training[47,48,51] • Removes need for urban simulation technicians and equipment or subspecialty content experts to travel to rural areas for in situ simulation training[47,48,51] • Increases the frequency rural clinicians deliberately practice neonatal and pediatric clinical scenarios rarely encountered[46,49,51,52] • Increasing frequency of training helps maintain skills (previous studies demonstrate skills improve immediately following simulation training, but there is a decline without regular repeated training sessions[53–56]) • Aligns with ILCOR and AHA recommendation of frequent simulation sessions to optimize skill retention[57]
Performance improvement	• Feasible and acceptable and improves performance similar to in-person simulation[21,48,50,58,59] • Excellent interrater reliability between in situ and remote simulation educators[60] • Similar learning outcomes and higher procedural performance scores following telesimulation training as compared with in situ training[61]
Realistic scenarios with real-time feedback	• Allows for tailored scenarios to address the challenges faced by rural teams • Provides opportunities to practice procedural skills and receive real-time feedback from trained pediatric simulation or subspecialist facilitators during the debriefing session[46,47] • Increases collaboration between rural and urban teams for professional development, maintenance of evidence-based knowledge, and procedural skills[46,48,51,62]
Affordability	• Lack of formal cost analyses of simulation programs, including ongoing costs associated with simulation training (eg, program coordination and clinician time)[63] • Elimination of travel expenses and the opportunity cost for participants' time away from clinical activities results in a cost reduction as compared with mobile simulation programs
Team-based training	• Allows scenario practice in an immersive interprofessional team environment • Demonstrated feasibility of team training and improvement in knowledge of current neonatal resuscitation guidelines with medical students and neonatal nurses[50] • Improvement in simulated and real patient outcomes with telesimulation programs teaching procedures[52] and critical care[64] cases globally in developing countries

and practice, rural clinicians lack opportunities for clinical exposure to HALO neonatal and pediatric emergencies. Increased training opportunities may not translate into consistent improvements in clinical outcomes and reduction in health care disparities.

Future directions of telesimulation

Future directions of telesimulation include enhanced technological innovations, such as virtual and augmented reality (AR), to enhance realism, accessibility, and

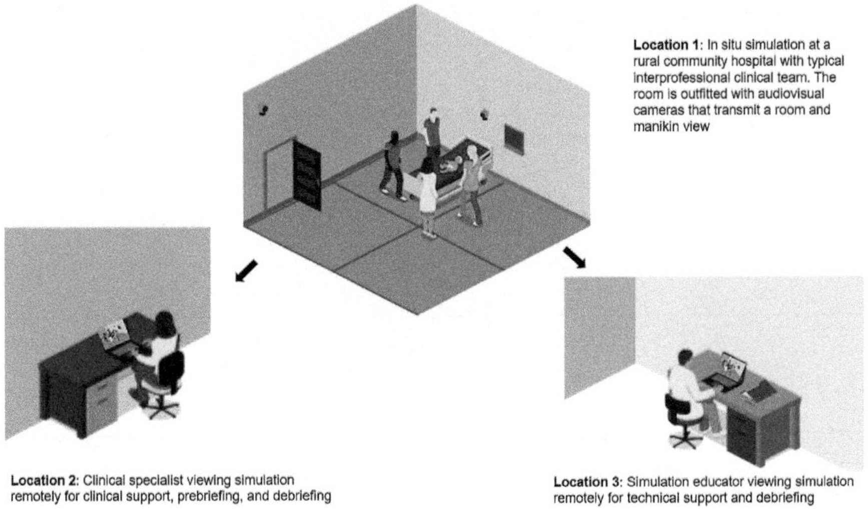
Location 1: In situ simulation at a rural community hospital with typical interprofessional clinical team. The room is outfitted with audiovisual cameras that transmit a room and manikin view
Location 2: Clinical specialist viewing simulation remotely for clinical support, prebriefing, and debriefing
Location 3: Simulation educator viewing simulation remotely for technical support and debriefing

Fig. 3. Telesimulation setup.

cost-effectiveness.[46,49] Additional work is needed to evaluate low-cost options for telesimulation, such as phone cameras or tablets for streaming. Information sharing and collaboration between the expanding telesimulation programs across rural and global areas create the ability to reduce the implementation burden[46] and facilitate further growth. Distance simulation programs may also allow the practice and implementation of real-patient telehealth programs to create a comprehensive approach to the care of pediatric patients in rural environments. These distance telehealth options may synergically improve clinical outcomes, health care team satisfaction, and retention[51] in underserved areas.

Extended Reality

The term extended reality (XR) is used for technologies that enhance or replace our view of the world. XR encompasses 3 different modalities: virtual reality (VR), AR, and mixed reality (MR). XR is increasingly being used to enhance Hi-Fi simulation.

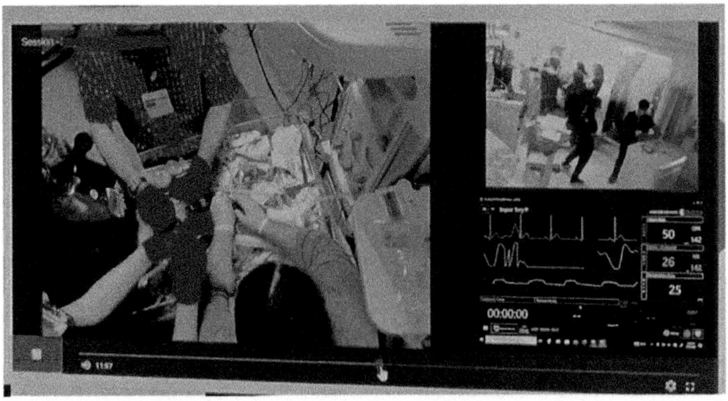

Fig. 4. Telesimulation views for remote specialists: room view, manikin view, and monitor view.

Hi-Fi simulation uses sophisticated manikins designed to authentically mimic the patient's appearance, sounds, and physiologic responses. Although there have been advances in the fidelity of lung and cardiac sounds, other clinical examination findings, such as skin appearance, including perfusion, rashes, pallor, and cyanosis, as well as aspects of the neurologic examination, such as mental status, tone, and movements, have lagged behind. XR realistically portrays these additional visual cues, which are critical to assessing the patient's clinical status. In VR, the learner wears a headset that isolates them from their surroundings, creating an entirely synthetic world where the environment, including equipment, manikins, and interventions, are animated. Alternatively, AR places holographic images within a real-world setting. Sophisticated holograms can be projected using specialized headsets with transparent lenses through which participants see a holographic, three-dimensional image in their actual space. In MR simulation, the hologram can be projected onto a manikin, and its physical and physiologic features can change based on the participants' actions. This section focuses on the advantages and disadvantages of VR, AR, and MR simulation (**Table 3**).

Implementation of extended reality simulation

In its simplest form, each learner only needs a headset with a software program to use XR technology (**Fig. 5**). In recent years, there has been a focus on using VR in medical education, particularly for training in lower-resource, rural environments.[67] VR does not require a dedicated simulation space, and training can be done asynchronously from any location. To further improve the fidelity of the scenario, haptic feedback devices can be paired with the XR technology. AR is a newer modality, but the setup requirements are quite similar. Like VR, AR does not require a dedicated space; however, the hologram can be projected in the in situ environment to significantly increase fidelity. All team members with a headset will see each other and the hologram, maximizing the opportunity for team training. The hologram can be projected over a physical manikin, creating an MR simulation. An advantage of MR is that all standard clinical equipment

Table 3
Comparison of extended reality technologies

Technology	Augmented Reality/ Mixed Reality	Virtual Reality
Equipment	• Headsets • Clinical equipment • Manikin • Software	• Headsets only • Optional haptic feedback devices • Software
Location	In situ or simulation center	Does not require dedicated space
Individual or team-based use	Individual or team-based *All team members can be present and participate*	Individual (limited team) *Option for team members to participate in avatar form*
Fidelity	High • The hologram can be placed over a manikin • All standard clinical equipment can be used and procedures performed	Low • Animated room and equipment • Haptic feedback devices can be used to increase fidelity
Average costs of headsets	~$3000	~$500

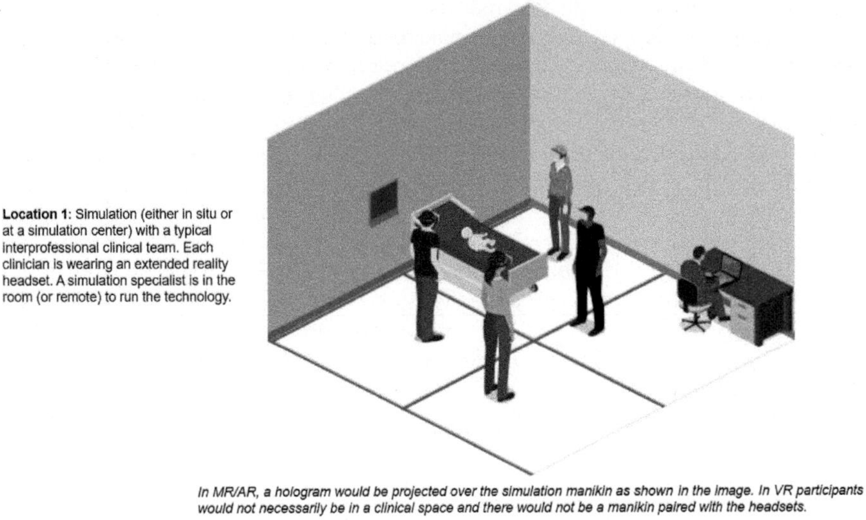
Location 1: Simulation (either in situ or at a simulation center) with a typical interprofessional clinical team. Each clinician is wearing an extended reality headset. A simulation specialist is in the room (or remote) to run the technology.
In MR/AR, a hologram would be projected over the simulation manikin as shown in the image. In VR participants would not necessarily be in a clinical space and there would not be a manikin paired with the headsets.

Fig. 5. ER simulation setup example.

can be used by team members to perform procedures on the manikin during the simulations. In MR, participants can experience increased authenticity of the scenario as the hologram can depict AV changes in physical examination and physiologic parameters. As a result of these advanced clinical states, a lower-cost, less-sophisticated manikin can be used in trainings without losing the AV feedback and providing opportunity to enhance feedback beyond the capabilities of a Hi-Fi manikin.

Benefits of extended reality

Although VR technology has activation costs, it is much more affordable than establishing a Hi-Fi laboratory, which has start-up costs in excess of $250,000.[68] VR cases have already been created and marketed for a variety of medical education implementations: scoliosis surgery,[69] endovascular neurosurgery,[70] hip surgery,[71] urinary catheterization,[72] laparoscopic surgery[72] (Zhengqian), and to practice engaging in difficult patient conversations.[73] VR scenarios have also been studied in pediatric emergency department resuscitation[74] (Willett, Chang). Similarly, AR has now been used to assist in adult advanced life support training,[75] anatomy education,[76] neurosurgery,[77] laparoscopic surgery,[78] and jaundice recognition[72] (Anderson). In the laparoscopic study, AR was shown to be superior to VR in realism, haptic feedback, and perceived usefulness. MR, therefore, offers the potential for optimizing team training in rural areas at a lower cost than Hi-Fi simulation.[79] The MR software can be designed to allow learners to program their own scenarios, or alternatively, content experts can preprogram high-yield scenarios. The response of the hologram can also be adjusted based on participant actions, rather than being preprogrammed according to an algorithm. The resuscitation training can be delivered to the entire resuscitation team, each wearing a lens to see and hear the same hologram simultaneously, with an opportunity for hands-on training using the equipment and interprofessional team members that would be available for an actual resuscitation.[80]

Limitations of extended reality

Despite the possibilities that XR technologies offer to enhance simulation, each technology poses varying limitations when used for medical education (**Table 4**). A

Table 4
Comparison of extended reality modalities

	Extended Reality	
Characteristics	**Virtual Reality**	**Mixed Reality/ Augmented Reality**
Patient fidelity	Low	High
Home environment fidelity	Low	High
Skill training fidelity	Low	High
Affordability	High	Medium
Portability	High	High
Acceptability	Medium	Medium
Familiarity	Medium	Low
Team training	Low	High
Capability for experts to join remotely	Low	Variable

disadvantage of VR compared with Hi-Fi simulation is that equipment and muscle movements used to resuscitate in a virtual environment are also virtual. Although it may increase access to training and help the individual learner refresh their knowledge, VR may not be sufficient for team-based hands-on skill acquisition or maintenance[81,82] and may be inferior to low-fidelity simulation training in skill-based scenarios.[82] Complicating matters, a meta-analysis of all XR modalities did not show any proven benefit in terms of skill acquisition or efficiency but did show some benefit in terms of user confidence.[83]

In most existing VR simulations, participants are not training in their native environment nor synchronously with their interprofessional team. There exists the technological capacity to create three-dimensional images of real environments in order to create an animated VR representation of a team's clinical base; however, these are not readily commercially available. Most existing VR educational tools are also individual and asynchronous. Efforts have been made to create shared-simulation models to improve interdisciplinary aspects[72] (DeBitetto); however, participants interact with animated avatars of each other rather than the humans themselves, and nonverbal communication is lost.

Side effects are also a problem with some users of XR headsets. VR technologies have the most reported side effects from usage when compared with other XR technologies. One study found participants commonly complained of headaches (25%), dizziness (40%), and blurred vision (35%).[84] AR technologies have fewer reported side effects and offer increased realism but are more expensive.

Although individual headsets are less expensive than a Hi-Fi simulation setup, in order to achieve optimal team training in XR simulation, each participant must wear individual headsets, thus multiplying costs.

Future directions of extended reality

XR provides opportunities for training at a Hi-Fi level, with lower costs than traditional Hi-Fi manikin training. This is even more important in areas where simulation may not have been previously possible at all. AR headsets allow experts to join the simulation remotely, observing performance and giving feedback to participants, thus bringing real-time expertise to rural areas. The ultimate goal of XR simulation is to simulate an environment that induces the stress of a real-life scenario, create a realistic depiction that will make the learner feel an empathetic desire to help their animated patient, work within an environment that is physically very similar to their own work environment, perform tasks that invoke the muscle memory needed for clinical tasks, and share this experience with the same interprofessional team used in real-life scenarios.

Many of these goals are achieved by using MR because the headsets are clear and the learner can use them in their home environment. A neonatal resuscitation model using a VR simulator with a manikin for tactile interactions was recently developed.[85] Although this can be considered an MR simulator, it uses VR headsets as the primary image source, forcing the participant to practice the simulation in a fully animated environment. Unless the native clinical layout can be replicated by partnering with a VR software developer at a significant cost, the virtual environment is generic. Although Zackoff and colleagues[86] demonstrated the ability to enhance the appearance of shock using an MR hologram overlaying a Hi-Fi manikin, it is fair to say that utilization of MR technology in simulations merits further study and development.[87] Despite the emerging technology, few medical MR prototypes exist, and acceptability and performance remain unknown compared with traditional Hi-Fi manikins. The authors are currently refining an MR neonatal resuscitation prototype (**Fig. 6**) that uses AR headsets and a hologram of a moving, breathing patient to be projected over a low-fidelity manikin[74] (Ferguson).

In the general public, XR devices have begun to gain acceptance, particularly in the gaming community. Despite this acceptance, XR technologies do create an increased cognitive load for new users and can pose challenges for individuals who are slower to adopt to new technology. Introductory training in the technology is thus necessary to increase participant comfort and ease of use. Information technology support at simulation sites have to acquire expertise in these XR technologies to support simulation sessions and onboarding of new learners to the devices. VR and AR technologies offer an exciting glimpse into the future of simulation; to be used regularly for medical education, the technology requires increased familiarity and decreased cognitive load.

DISCUSSION

As rural pediatric and maternity inpatient units continue to close across the United States, supporting rural clinicians by providing state-of-the-art, regular training opportunities to care for pediatric patients is essential. Continued education to practice HALO events is vital for rural clinicians to maintain skills and be prepared for events. Traditional simulation programs are resource-intensive and often inaccessible to smaller hospitals that do not have the financial means to purchase necessary simulation equipment nor have subspecialists or simulation experts at their sites. To address

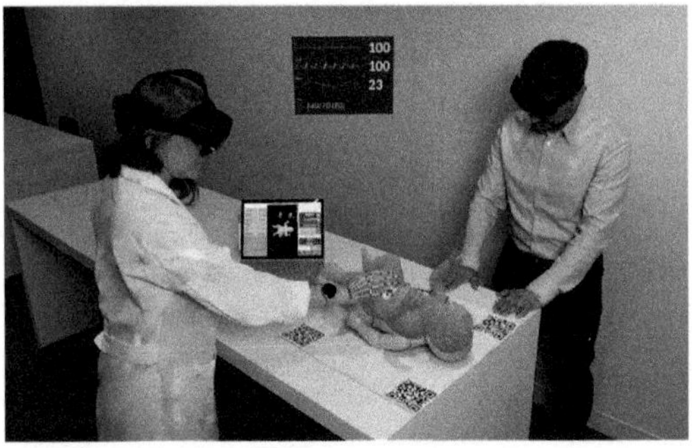

Fig. 6. Example of mixed reality neonatal prototype.

this, nationwide researchers have identified novel alternatives to traditional simulation, including telesimulation, mobile simulation, and ER simulation. These modalities address barriers of geographic distance, access to specialized expertise, affordability, and access. Although many barriers are addressed, these modalities have limitations, including availability and accessibility, user acceptance, and technology expertise. In addition, stakeholder support, protected time for clinicians to participate, and local champions to coordinate sessions are needed for simulation training to be successful. Further research is needed to study how these technologies, such as distance simulation and ER, compare with traditional simulation to make these novel approaches accessible to all rural hospitals, including those not affiliated with a larger academic institution.

SUMMARY

Although simulation is effective in various areas, including team confidence, procedural skills, and patient safety, there exists a paucity of information on how simulation training translates to patient outcomes. Additional multicenter studies are needed to assess the impact on pediatric morbidity and mortality. By using mobile simulation, telesimulation, and ER, rural health care providers can access effective and regular training opportunities to remain ready to respond to HALO events.

CLINICS CARE POINTS

- Innovative technologies such as mobile simulation, telesimulation, and extended reality offer rural clinicians enhanced access to vital simulation training, bridging the gap between rural and urbal health care quality particularly for high-acuity, low-occurence (HALO) events.
- Regular reinforcement of HALO events through repeated simulation sessions is crucial for retaining proficiency and improving patient outcomes.
- Telesimulation provides a cost-effective alternative to traditional in-person simulation training by removing the need for clinicians to travel and reducing the logistical burden on rural hospitals, enabling frequent practice sessions, critical for maintaining skills in low-resource settings.
- Simulation training fosters collaboration between rural hospitals and larger academic centers leading to significant improvements in pediatric readiness and overall patient safety.

DISCLOSURE

Drs M. Ferguson, M. Melendi, M. Ottolini and A. Zanno are co-developers (with Case Western Reserve) of a mixed reality neonatal prototype, HoloBaby, that is not yet commercially available. All authors have no conflicts of interest, and there are no relevant funding disclosures to report.

REFERENCES

1. Bettenhausen JL, Winterer CM, Colvin JD. Health and poverty of rural children: an under-researched and under-resourced vulnerable population. Academic Pediatrics 2021;21(8, Supplement):S126–33.
2. Dugani SB, Hubach RD. Equity, multisector collaboration and innovation for rural health: lessons from the National Rural Health Association Conference. Rural Remote Health 2023;23(2):8485.

3. Ames SG, Davis BS, Marin JR, et al. Emergency department pediatric readiness and mortality in critically ill children. Pediatrics 2019;144(3). https://doi.org/10.1542/peds.2019-0568.
4. Newgard CD, Lin A, Goldhaber-Fiebert JD, et al, Pediatric Readiness Study Group. Association of emergency department pediatric readiness with mortality to 1 year among injured children treated at trauma centers. JAMA Surg 2022;157(4):e217419.
5. Michelson KA, Hudgins JD, Monuteaux MC, et al. Cardiac arrest survival in pediatric and general emergency departments. Pediatrics 2018;141(2).
6. Larson KCW, Racine AD, Racine AD, et al. Trends in access to health care services for US children: 2000-2014. Pediatrics 2016;138:e20162176.
7. Marcin JP, Shaikh U, Steinhorn RH. Addressing health disparities in rural communities using telehealth. Pediatr Res 2016;79(1):169–76.
8. Cushing AM, Bucholz EM, Chien AT, et al. Availability of pediatric inpatient services in the United States. Pediatrics 2021;148(1). e2020041723.
9. VonAchen P, Davis MM, Cartland J, et al. Closure of licensed pediatric beds in health care markets within Illinois. Acad Pediatr 2022;22(3):431–9.
10. Leyenaar JK, Freyleue SD, Arakelyan M, et al. Pediatric hospitalizations at rural and urban teaching and nonteaching hospitals in the US, 2009-2019. JAMA Netw Open 2023;6(9):e2331807. PMID: 37656457; PMCID: PMC10474556.
11. Iyer MS, Way DP, Schumacher DJ, et al. How general pediatricians learn procedures: implications for training and practice. Med Educ Online 2021;26(1):1985935.
12. Lieng MK, Marcin JP, Sigal IS, et al. Association between emergency department pediatric readiness and transfer of noninjured children in small rural hospitals. J Rural Health 2022;38(1):293–302.
13. Abulebda K, Whitfill T, Montgomery EE, et al. Improving pediatric readiness in general emergency departments: a prospective interventional study. J Pediatr 2021;230:230–7.e1.
14. Ericsson KA. Deliberate practice and acquisition of expert performance: a general overview. Acad Emerg Med 2008;15(11):988–94.
15. Wang JM, Zorek JA. Deliberate practice as a theoretical framework for interprofessional experiential education. Front Pharmacol 2016;7:188.
16. Yousef N, Moreau R, Soghier L. Simulation in neonatal care: towards a change in traditional training? Eur J Pediatr 2022;181(4):1429–36.
17. Bhanji F, Finn JC, Lockey A, et al. Part 8: Education, implementation, and teams: 2015 international consensus on cardiopulmonary resuscitation and emergency cardiovascular care science with treatment recommendations. Circulation 2015;132(16 Suppl 1):S242–68.
18. Ackermann AD, Kenny G, Walker C. Simulator programs for new nurses' orientation: a retention strategy. J Nurses Staff Dev 2007;23(3):136–9.
19. Baik D, Zierler BRN. Job Satisfaction and Retention After an Interprofessional Team Intervention. West J Nurs Res 2019;41.
20. Al Sabei SD, Labrague LJ, Al-Rawajfah O, et al. Relationship between interprofessional teamwork and nurses' intent to leave work: The mediating role of job satisfaction and burnout. Nurs Forum 2022;57(4):568–76.
21. Harper MG, Bodine J, Monachino A. The effectiveness of simulation use in transition to practice nurse residency programs: a review of literature from 2009 to 2018. Journal for Nurses in Professional Development 2021;37(6).

22. Janes G, Mills T, Budworth L, et al. The association between health care staff engagement and patient safety outcomes: a systematic review and meta-analysis. J Patient Saf 2021;17(3):207–16.
23. Mileder LP, Schmölzer GM. Simulation-based training: the missing link to lastingly improved patient safety and health? Postgrad Med J 2016;92(1088):309–11.
24. Kharasch M, Aitchison P, Ochoa P, et al. Growth of a simulation lab: engaging the learner is key to success. Disease-a-Month 2011;57(11):679–90.
25. Healthcare Simulation Dictionary, Society for Simulation in Healthcare. Available at: https://www.ssih.org/Dictionary.
26. Guise L. Mobile sim lab helps medical professionals save lives. 2024. Available at: https://info.lifelinemobile.com/blog/mobile-sim-labs-help-medical-professionals-save-lives.
27. Singhal N, Lockyer J, Fidler H, et al. Helping Babies Breathe: global neonatal resuscitation program development and formative educational evaluation. Resuscitation 2012;83(1):90–6.
28. Arlington L, Kairuki AK, Isangula KG, et al. Implementation of "Helping Babies Breathe": A 3-Year Experience in Tanzania. Pediatrics 2017;139(5). https://doi.org/10.1542/peds.2016-2132.
29. Msemo G, Massawe A, Mmbando D, et al. Newborn mortality and fresh stillbirth rates in Tanzania after helping babies breathe training. Pediatrics 2013;131(2): e353–60.
30. Bellad RM, Bang A, Carlo WA, et al. A pre-post study of a multi-country scale up of resuscitation training of facility birth attendants: does Helping Babies Breathe training save lives? BMC Pregnancy Childbirth 2016;16(1):222.
31. Ersdal H, Vossius C, Bayo E, et al. A one-day "helping babies breathe" course improves simulated performance but not clinical management of neonates. Resuscitation 2013;84. https://doi.org/10.1016/j.resuscitation.2013.04.005.
32. Dol Justine, Campbell-Yeo Marsha, Murphy Gail Tomblin, et al. The impact of the Helping Babies Survive program on neonatal outcomes and health provider skills: a systematic review. JBI Database of Systematic Reviews and Implementation Reports 2018;16(3):701–37.
33. Legoux C, Gerein R, Boutis K, et al. Retention of critical procedural skills after simulation training: a systematic review. AEM Educ Train 2021;5(3):e10536.
34. Ansquer R, Mesnier T, Farampour F, et al. Long-term retention assessment after simulation-based-training of pediatric procedural skills among adult emergency physicians: a multicenter observational study. BMC Med Educ 2019;19(1):348.
35. Brazil V. Translational simulation: not 'where?' but 'why?' A functional view of in situ simulation. Advances in Simulation 2017;2(1):20.
36. Abulebda K, Lutfi R, Whitfill T, et al. A Collaborative In Situ Simulation-based Pediatric Readiness Improvement Program for Community Emergency Departments. Acad Emerg Med 2018;25(2):177–85.
37. Mitchell SA, Boyer TJ. Deliberate practice in medical simulation. *StatPearls*. StatPearls Publishing Copyright © 2024, StatPearls Publishing LLC.; 2024.
38. Riaz S. How simulation-based medical education can be started in low resource settings. J Ayub Med Coll Abbottabad 2019;31(4):636–7. PMID: 31933328.
39. Raemer D, Hannenberg A, Mullen A. Simulation safety first: an imperative. Simul Healthc 2018;13(6):373–5.
40. Raemer DB. Ignaz Semmelweis redux? Simul Healthc. 2014;9(3):153–5.
41. Raemer D, Hannenberg A, Mullen A. Simulation safety first: an imperative. Adv Simul (Lond). 2018;3:25.

42. Tyng CM, Amin HU, Saad MNM, et al. The influences of emotion on learning and memory. Front Psychol 2017;8:1454.
43. Norman J. Systematic review of the literature on simulation in nursing education. Abnf j. Spring 2012;23(2):24–8.
44. Nippita S, Haviland MJ, Voit SF, et al. Randomized trial of high- and low-fidelity simulation to teach intrauterine contraception placement. Am J Obstet Gynecol 2018;218(2):258.e1–11.
45. Finan E, Bismilla Z, Whyte HE, et al. High-fidelity simulator technology may not be superior to traditional low-fidelity equipment for neonatal resuscitation training. J Perinatol 2012;32(4):287–92.
46. Fang JL, Umoren RA. Telesimulation for neonatal resuscitation training. Semin Perinatol 2023;47(7):151827.
47. McCoy CE, Sayegh J, Alrabah R, et al. Telesimulation: An Innovative Tool for Health Professions Education. AEM Educ Train 2017;1(2):132–6.
48. Honda R, McCoy CE. Teledebriefing in medical simulation, . StatPearls. Treasure Island, FL: StatPearls Publishing LLC; 2024.
49. Yasser NBM, Tan AJQ, Harder N, et al. Telesimulation in healthcare education: A scoping review. Nurse Educ Today 2023;126:105805.
50. Mileder LP, Bereiter M, Wegscheider T. Telesimulation as a modality for neonatal resuscitation training. Med Educ Online 2021;26(1):1892017.
51. Donohue LT, Hoffman KR, Marcin JP. Use of Telemedicine to Improve Neonatal Resuscitation. Children 2019;6(4). https://doi.org/10.3390/children6040050.
52. Mikrogianakis A, Kam A, Silver S, et al. Telesimulation: an innovative and effective tool for teaching novel intraosseous insertion techniques in developing countries. Acad Emerg Med 2011;18(4):420–7.
53. Trevisanuto D, Ferrarese P, Cavicchioli P, et al. Knowledge gained by pediatric residents after neonatal resuscitation program courses. Paediatr Anaesth 2005; 15(11):944–7.
54. Matterson HH, Szyld D, Green BR, et al. Neonatal resuscitation experience curves: simulation based mastery learning booster sessions and skill decay patterns among pediatric residents. J Perinat Med 2018;46(8):934–41.
55. Patel J, Posencheg M, Ades A. Proficiency and retention of neonatal resuscitation skills by pediatric residents. Pediatrics 2012;130(3):515–21.
56. Bender J, Kennally K, Shields R, et al. Does simulation booster impact retention of resuscitation procedural skills and teamwork? J Perinatol 2014;34(9):664–8.
57. Bhanji F, Finn JC, Lockey A, et al. Part 8: Education, Implementation, and Teams: 2015 International Consensus on Cardiopulmonary Resuscitation and Emergency Cardiovascular Care Science With Treatment Recommendations. Circulation 2015;132(16 Suppl 1):S242–68.
58. Naik N, Finkelstein RA, Howell J, et al. Telesimulation for COVID-19 Ventilator Management Training With Social-Distancing Restrictions During the Coronavirus Pandemic. Simulat Gaming 2020;51(4):571–7.
59. Hughes M, Gerstner B, Bona A, et al. Adaptive change in simulation education: comparison of effectiveness of a communication skill curriculum on death notification using in person methods versus a digital communication platform. AEM Educ Train 2021;5(3):e10610.
60. Okrainec A, Vassiliou M, Kapoor A, et al. Feasibility of remote administration of the Fundamentals of Laparoscopic Surgery (FLS) skills test. Surg Endosc 2013;27(11):4033–7.

61. Jewer J, Parsons MH, Dunne C, et al. Evaluation of a mobile telesimulation unit to train rural and remote practitioners on high-acuity low-occurrence procedures: pilot randomized controlled trial. J Med Internet Res 2019;21(8):e14587.
62. Hayden EM, Khatri A, Kelly HR, et al. Mannequin-based Telesimulation: Increasing Access to Simulation-based Education. Acad Emerg Med 2018; 25(2):144–7.
63. Hippe DS, Umoren RA, McGee A, et al. A targeted systematic review of cost analyses for implementation of simulation-based education in healthcare. SAGE Open Med 2020;8. 2050312120913451.
64. James EJG, Vyasam S, Venkatachalam S, et al. Low-cost "telesimulation" training improves real patient pediatric shock outcomes in India. Front Pediatr 2022 Jul 26;10:904846.
65. Doucette EJ, Fullerton MM, Pateman M, et al. Development and evaluation of virtual simulation games to increase the confidence and self-efficacy of healthcare learners in vaccine communication, advocacy, and promotion. BMC Med Educ 2024;24(1):190.
66. Bajwa M, Ahmed R, Lababidi H, et al. Development of Distance Simulation Educator Guidelines in Healthcare: A Delphi Method Application. Simul Healthc 2024;19(1):1–10.
67. Ghoman SK, Patel SD, Cutumisu M, et al. Serious games, a game changer in teaching neonatal resuscitation? A review. Arch Dis Child Fetal Neonatal Ed 2020;105(1):98–107.
68. Kharasch M, Aitchison P, Ochoa P, et al. Growth of a simulation lab: engaging the learner is key to success. Dis Mon 2011;57(11):679–90.
69. Izard SG, Juanes JA, García Peñalvo FJ, et al. Virtual reality as an educational and training tool for medicine. J Med Syst 2018;42(3):50.
70. Fargen KM, Siddiqui AH, Veznedaroglu E, et al. Simulator based angiography education in neurosurgery: results of a pilot educational program. J Neurointerv Surg 2012;4(6):438–41.
71. Sun P, Zhao Y, Men J, et al. Application of virtual and augmented reality technology in hip surgery: systematic review. J Med Internet Res 2023;25:e37599.
72. Abstracts Presented at the 24th Annual International Meeting on Simulation in Healthcare, January 20–24, 2024, San Diego, CA. Simulat Healthc J Soc Med Simulat 2024;19(1):e1–51. https://doi.org/10.1097/sih.0000000000000778.
73. Kuehn BM. Virtual and augmented reality put a twist on medical education. JAMA 2018;319(8):756–8.
74. Abstracts Presented at the 23rd Annual International Meeting on Simulation in Healthcare, January 21–25, 2023, Orlando, FL. Simulat Healthc J Soc Med Simulat 2023;18(3):e1–42. https://doi.org/10.1097/sih.0000000000000731.
75. Komasawa N, Ohashi T, Take A, et al. Hybrid simulation training utilizing augmented reality and simulator for interprofessional advanced life support training. J Clin Anesth 2019;57:106–7.
76. Ma M, Fallavollita P, Seelbach I, et al. Personalized augmented reality for anatomy education. Clin Anat 2016;29(4):446–53.
77. Cho J, Rahimpour S, Cutler A, et al. Enhancing reality: a systematic review of augmented reality in neuronavigation and education. World Neurosurg 2020; 139:186–95.
78. Botden SM, Buzink SN, Schijven MP, et al. Augmented versus virtual reality laparoscopic simulation: what is the difference? A comparison of the ProMIS augmented reality laparoscopic simulator versus LapSim virtual reality laparoscopic simulator. World J Surg 2007;31(4):764–72.

79. Yilmaz R. Educational magic toys developed with augmented reality technology for early childhood education. Comput Hum Behav 2016;54:240–8.
80. Abstracts Presented at the 24th Annual International Meeting on Simulation in Healthcare, January 20–24, 2024, San Diego, CA. Simulation in Healthcare. The Journal of the Society for Simulation in Healthcare 2024;19(1):e1–51.
81. Mitha AP, Almekhlafi MA, Janjua MJ, et al. Simulation and augmented reality in endovascular neurosurgery: lessons from aviation. Neurosurgery 2013; 72(Suppl 1):107–14.
82. Scerbo MW, Schmidt EA, Bliss JP. Comparison of a virtual reality simulator and simulated limbs for phlebotomy training. J Infus Nurs 2006;29(4):214–24.
83. Maheu-Cadotte MA, Cossette S, Dubé V, et al. Efficacy of serious games in healthcare professions education: a systematic review and meta-analysis. Simul Healthc 2021;16(3):199–212.
84. Moro C, Štromberga Z, Raikos A, et al. The effectiveness of virtual and augmented reality in health sciences and medical anatomy. Anat Sci Educ 2017;10(6):549–59.
85. Coduri M, Calandrino A, Addiego Mobilio G, et al. A mixed reality simulator for newborn life support training. PLoS One 2023;18(12):e0294914.
86. Zackoff MW, Cruse B, Sahay RD, et al. Development and implementation of augmented reality enhanced high-fidelity simulation for recognition of patient decompensation. Simul Healthc 2021;16(3):221–30.
87. Gerup J, Soerensen CB, Dieckmann P. Augmented reality and mixed reality for healthcare education beyond surgery: an integrative review. Int J Med Educ 2020;11:1–18.

Preparing Residents for Rural Practice and Advocacy

The Experiences of Three Residency Training Programs in the Northeast United States (2009–2023)

Brian Youth, MD[a,b,*], Carol Lynn O'Dea, MD[c,1], Jill Rinehart, MD[d,2]

KEYWORDS

• Rural • Residency training • Community • Advocacy • Underserved

KEY POINTS

- Pediatric residency training with embedded rural medicine experiences in a rural setting provides trainees with unique experiences and increases the number of trainees practicing in a rural setting after graduation.
- Pediatric residency training in a rural setting prepares trainees for pediatric subspecialty fellowship training, and resident graduates from rural training programs continue to choose pediatric subspecialty training despite overall declining numbers applying to pediatric subspecialty fellowship training nationally.
- Rural medicine education and exposure in pediatric residency are inherently connected to advocacy training and provide excellent opportunities for pediatric residency projects as well as collaboration between pediatric residency programs.

INTRODUCTION

Training providers to work in rural settings has never been more important than it is today. As pathway programs are considered that expose both medical students

[a] Department of Pediatrics, Tufts University School of Medicine, Boston, MA, USA; [b] Pediatric Residency, Maine Medical Center, The Barbara Bush Children's Hospital at Maine Medical Center, 22 Bramhall Street, Portland, ME 04101, USA; [c] Department of Pediatrics, Pediatric Residency, Children's Hospital at Dartmouth–Hitchcock/Geisel School of Medicine, 1 Medical Center Drive, Lebanon, NH 03756, USA; [d] Department of Pediatrics, Robert J. Larner College of Medicine at the University of Vermont, Pediatric Residency Program, University of Vermont Children's Hospital, 111 Colchester Avenue, Burlington, VT 05401, USA
[1] Present address: 39 Rayton Road, Hanover, NH 03755.
[2] Present address: 38 Madison Drive, Williston, VT 05495.
* Corresponding author. MaineHealth- Pediatric and Internal Medicine Clinic- Portland, Maine Medical Center, 22 Bramhall Street, Portland, ME 04101.
E-mail address: Brian.Youth@mainehealth.org

Pediatr Clin N Am 72 (2025) 151–164
https://doi.org/10.1016/j.pcl.2024.07.029 pediatric.theclinics.com

and residents to rural medicine, it is important to keep in mind some dire facts. As noted in the *AAMC News*,[1] of the more than 7200 federally designated health professional shortage areas, 60% are in rural regions, and although 20% of the US population lives in rural communities, only 11% of physicians practice in such areas. The lack of physicians is deeply worrisome. That is in part because rural residents are more likely to die of health issues like cardiovascular disease, unintentional injury, and chronic lung disease than city-dwellers. Rural residents also tend to be diagnosed with cancer at later stages and have worse outcomes. This situation will clearly worsen as many rural physicians near retirement; nearly a quarter fewer may be practicing by 2030.[2]

Equally troubling, medical school matriculants from rural areas—who are most likely to practice in such regions—declined 28% between 2002 and 2017, reports a 2019 study led by Scott Shipman, MD, AAMC,[3] director of primary care initiatives and clinical innovations, and that decline came at a time when the overall number of matriculants increased by 30%.

Many studies have looked at factors that lead medical students to consider careers in rural medicine after training. A recent *British Medical Journal* article[4] found that even short-term (12 weeks) placement in a rural setting during medical school training positively influenced future practice in rural communities. Another study that evaluated the rural exposure in training to residents from a family medicine training program found a linear gradient between time spent in rural settings during residency and subsequent rural practice.[5]

Elma and colleagues[6] noted that physician maldistribution is a global problem that hinders patients' abilities to access health care services. They go on to state that medial education presents an opportunity to influence physicians toward meeting the health care needs of underserved communities when establishing their practice and identifies several factors that educators be mindful of in choosing medical students. Some of these factors include consideration for rural experiences during undergraduate and postgraduate medical training, the value of financial incentives, and better understanding the motivations of aspiring physicians, noting that these motivations have considerable impact on the effectiveness of education initiatives designed to influence physician distribution to underserved locations.

The Accreditation Council for Graduate Medical Education (ACGME) along with other higher education organizations has over time moved away from using standardized test scores, grades in core clerkships, and even downplaying letters of recommendation in an effort to give medical students a more holistic review when choosing candidates for residency. Many programs are looking hard at their mission and seeking out candidates that meet that mission more fully by demonstrable past experience. A residency, the focus of which is on training primary care to fulfill an underserved workforce such as that that exists in rural communities, may be more likely to match a student who is from a rural background, or has spent time working in rural underserved settings.

Many institutions and medical schools have developed programs over the last decade with the goal of helping to increase the workforce of those entering rural practice. One of these programs at the University of North Carolina (UNC), School of Medicine is known as the "Fully Integrated Readiness for Service Training (FIRST) Program." This accelerated curriculum focused on rural and underserved care that links 3 years of medical school with a conditional acceptance into UNC's 3-year family medicine residency, followed by 3 years of practice support after graduation.[7] Students are recruited to the FIRST Program during the fall of their first year of medical school. The FIRST Program promotes close faculty mentorship and familiarity with the health care system, includes a longitudinal quality improvement project with an assigned patient panel, includes early integration into the clinic, and fosters a close cohort of fellow students. As of March 2020, the FIRST program had recruited 5 classes of medical students, and 3 of those classes had matched into residency—it remains to be seen as these classes finish their training how many of those students choose primary care in a rural setting as their postresidency path.

Clearly, pathway ideas meant to expose medical students (or even high school students) and residents to rural medicine may increase the numbers of those whom complete training and pursue rural medicine. Many larger residency programs have created rural "tracks" designed specifically to give interested students more time in rural communities with the belief that this will lead them to rural practice after training. Indeed, tying this training to guaranteed funding, loan relief, or opportunities for spousal employment will be beneficial in meeting the needs of the rural communities.

Longenecker and colleagues[8] recently published in the *Journal of Rural Health* some findings regarding the current landscape of rural efforts in US Undergraduate Medical Education (UME). This descriptive study of 182 allopathic and osteopathic medical schools found that few (only 8.2%) of them expressed an explicit commitment to producing rural physicians in public mission statements; however, most (64.8%) provided rural clinical experiences, and many demonstrated their commitment in other ways. It is important to note that of the two-thirds of programs that provided rural clinical experiences, only 39 (21%) did so through a formal rural program.

The American Academy of Pediatrics[9] (AAP) released the Pediatrician Workforce Policy Statement in 2013 with the conclusion that the "current distribution of primary care pediatricians is inadequate to meet the needs of children living in rural and other underserved areas." The statement also outlines that the shortage of pediatric subspecialists will disproportionately affect rural regions of the country.

The ACGME guidelines for Categorical Pediatrics are changing requirements such that beginning in July 2025, the required time trainees spend in critical care (both neonatal and pediatric) is reduced to 2 blocks of training. For those going into rural medicine, this may be inadequate to prepare residents for covering the delivery room and gaining necessary experience with stabilizing sick children before transport. With the changing ACGME recommendations, programs are committed to providing a focused experience to prepare pediatricians for rural practice, primarily by recommending self-directed elective choices in training that will benefit those who plan to practice in a rural environment. Examples of this curriculum are explained forthwith.

It is with the above in mind that the authors share how 3 pediatric training programs in the northeast that do not have a specified rural track have found success in populating rural communities with pediatricians. They also discuss how the residency programs allow for experiences and autonomy in residency that lead many to pursue posttraining fellowship programs, an added benefit given the workforce issues facing many communities in recruiting and retaining pediatric subspecialists. Finally, the authors briefly share a relatively new advocacy collaborative that brings residents together on a regular basis.

BACKGROUND

The pediatric residency programs of *The Barbara Bush Children's Hospital at Maine Medical Center*, the *Children's Hospital at Dartmouth–Hitchcock*, and the *University of Vermont Children's Hospital* all have long track records of training pediatricians that ultimately practice in a variety of settings. Like most training programs, each of these programs has decades of success producing pediatricians that go on for fellowship training, careers in academic medicine, or practicing primary care. What is unique about these 3 programs is that the exposure the authors provide for their learners, which includes dedicated, longitudinal time gaining a greater understanding of the practice of rural medicine, has led to many graduates choosing rural medicine either as a generalist or as a specialist as one's first practice experience after training (**Fig. 1**).

THE FOLLOWING IS A DETAILED DESCRIPTION OF THE RURAL CURRICULUM, EXPERIENCES, AND GRADUATE DATA FROM THESE THREE PROGRAMS.

The Barbara Bush Children's Hospital at Maine Medical Center

The pediatric residency program at Maine Medical Center (MMC) was first accredited in 1958. The program has graduated hundreds of residents over the ensuing decades, is the only pediatric training program in Maine, and is responsible for producing much of the state's primary care workforce as well as specialists. A significant number of the workforce that entered rural practice trained at MMC, and in the case of specialties, left Maine to pursue fellowship training and then came back to Maine to practice. The program does not have pediatric fellowships; yet, like many programs, 30% to 50% of graduates go on to complete fellowships at other institutions in any given year. Located in Portland, Maine, The Barbara Bush Children's Hospital is part of the larger MaineHealth Network that includes regional hospitals and primary care practices throughout Maine.

Approximately 61% of Mainers live in rural counties, and although most children in the state live in southern Maine, children of all ages and developmental stages live throughout the state and require access to high-quality pediatric care. In addition, the catchment area for The Barbara Bush Children's Hospital at Maine Medical Center is wide-ranging, inclusive of much of the State of Maine as well as parts of southern New Hampshire.

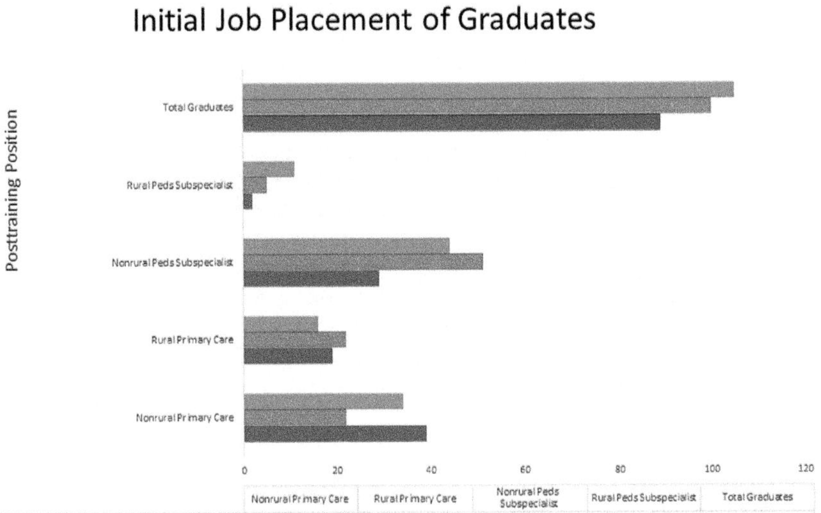

	Nonrural Primary Care	Rural Primary Care	Nonrural Peds Subspecialist	Rural Peds Subspecialist	Total Graduates
Children's Hospital at Dartmouth-Hitchcock	34	16	44	11	105
University of Vermont Children's Hospital	22	22	51	5	100
The Barbara Bush Children's Hospital at Maine Medical Center	39	19	29	2	89

Number of Residents

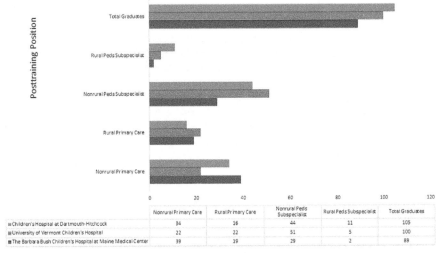

Fig. 1. Initial job placement of graduates (2009–2023).

MMC formalized a required rural rotation for all residents in 1997. The rural experience is a required block rotation for all interns and takes place between December and June of the intern year, so as to give learners time to first be acclimated to residency before embarking on time away from the medical center. Residents are placed in one of a growing number of rural practices, most of which are within 90 minutes of Portland, Maine. All communities have populations of less than 8000. From 1997 to 2008, there were 3 sites as the primary location for these learners. All 3 sites had pediatric faculty that were given Clinical Instructor status for their academic appointment with either the University of Vermont (medical school partner until 2010) or the Tufts University School of Medicine (2010 to current). In 2008, the authors expanded to a fourth site, and then in 2017, opened up their other affiliated MaineHealth pediatric practices throughout the state where faculty were eager to accept learners.

As the ACGME Pediatric Residency Review Committee requirements expanded to include 6 months of individualized training in 2012, the authors have had many residents choose a second or even third experience in a rural setting during the final 2 years of training. These experiences are optional for the learners.

The rural medicine curriculum is part of the authors' comprehensive ambulatory pediatric curriculum (**Box 1**), which includes several ambulatory rotations. The authors emphasize to learners that the curriculums for these various rotations should be viewed in a *continuum of learning* such that they are encouraged to make connections between the various experiences occurring in the different ambulatory experiences.

Thus, the authors' acute care pediatrics, continuity clinic, community pediatrics, rural medicine, and advocacy rotations all share a common curriculum and then have *specific competencies* that are met in the individual experiences, as depicted in **Box 1**. Although there are many shared competencies between these multiple

Box 1
The Barbara Bush Children's Hospital at Maine Medical Center Residency Program comprehensive ambulatory pediatric curriculum

Postgraduate Year (PGY-1)

- Acute Care Pediatrics—general pediatric resident clinic
- Continuity Clinics—dispersed throughout the year in "Y" block rotations
- Rural Pediatrics—4 weeks at one of the authors' affiliated rural sites (see addendum for curriculum)
- ACQUIRE—introduction to Advocacy, Community Pediatrics, QI, Research, and Education-
  - Block month designed to introduce all interns to these topics with goal of project initiation to continue into Advocacy year 2
  - Residents can select a rural-focused project of interest
  - Occurs as 2- to 2-week blocks—one in fall, one in spring

PGY-2 Year

- Continuity Clinics—dispersed throughout the year in "Y" block rotations
- Advocacy Rotation
  - Focused education on advocacy with a goal of completion of project from year 1
  - Exposure to statewide advocacy work highlighting the needs of urban and rural populations
- Community Pediatrics
  - Completed in a local practice under guidance of the authors' faculty
  - Can be in a rural site per resident choice

PGY-3 Year

- Continuity Clinics—dispersed throughout the year in "Y" block rotations
- Additional opportunities for Rural Exposure via Individualized Curricular Experiences

experiences, there are rotation-specific competencies unique to each experience as well. An example from the rural rotation may be "*to learn the role of the pediatrician as school health advisor*" or "*developing a care management plan for a child with complex health care needs*," which the authors found held more value for their residents when discussed on the rural rotation where primary care pediatricians are managing these patients with specialty consultation in a way that differs from practices that are co-located with specialists (as seen in the more urban centers of the state).

In terms of satisfaction with the rural rotation, resident and attending feedback has been strong. Residents note that they appreciated the complexity of primary care without tertiary care support, and the ability for greater community involvement (attending sports events as the team physician, participating in group sessions with adolescents, prenatal visits). They also note great satisfaction with the rural faculty with comments, such as "*I want to be a pediatrician just like Dr. X*" or "*Unbelievably devoted to pediatrics, teaching, and the community*."

Faculty also appreciate the opportunity to interact with resident learners noting comments, such as "*having residents provide a stimulus to stay up to date; the residents make me feel more connected to the tertiary medical center in Portland; and meeting the residents during the rural block makes it so nice when transferring sick patients to the inpatient services at the medical center.*"

Although exposure to rural primary care likely increases the workforce in this much needed area, what is also noteworthy is the feedback the authors receive from the graduates that pursue pediatric fellowships after training. Many patients in the region may present to critical access hospitals throughout the state, and the residents have the opportunity, with support from the pediatric critical care team, to participate in these transport calls and to be part of the transport team that goes out and brings these children back to MMC. For those entering procedural-based fellowships (neonatal intensive care unit [NICU], pediatric intensive care unit [PICU], cardiology), most note that they have had significantly more "hands-on" experience than many of their co-fellows that trained in larger programs with critically ill children. The authors think this is a direct result of training at their institutions where residents have the chance to participate in these transports and have more autonomy and direct patient care opportunities within their hospital services, as there are no fellows to share these procedures in training.

In terms of data over the last 15 years, the authors' program has graduated 89 residents; 65% pursued primary care or a non-fellowship hospitalist job after their training, and 35% pursued fellowship. **Fig. 2** depicts this as well as showing a split between rural and urban practice.

Of those that chose primary care, 16 of 43 residents (37%) chose to practice in a rural setting as their first job after residency. In addition, 3 residents joined practices primarily in a hospitalist role in a rural setting, but also do work in primary care. More importantly, 100% of those residents are either in that same first job or in a different practice that is still in a rural setting.

Of the 35% of residents that completed fellowship training (n = 31), the authors note that many of them now practice as a specialist in locations that serve children in rural areas. Although the authors' immediate community in Portland, Maine is not considered rural, 11 residents (35%) that completed fellowship in the last 15 years are now members of the authors' faculty and care for patients from both rural and urban areas at MMC.

University of Vermont Children's Hospital

The University of Vermont Children's Hospital pediatric residency program was first accredited in 1949 under the leadership of Dr Jim McKay, and since its inception

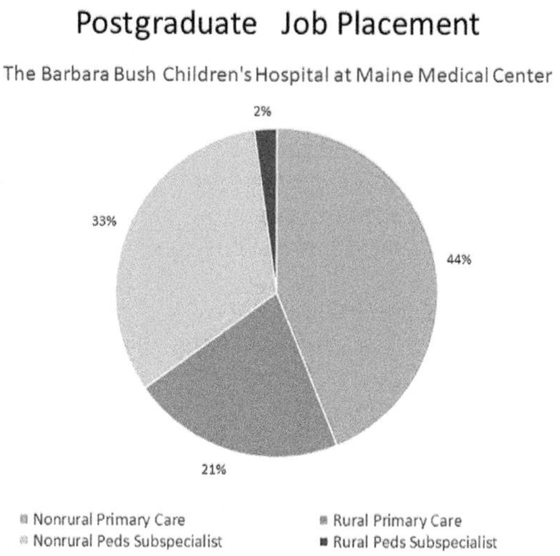

Fig. 2. The Barbara Bush Children's Hospital at Maine Medical Center pediatric residency program postgraduate job placement.

has been committed to maintaining a strong connection with community pediatricians throughout Vermont and upstate New York. This is evident in the commitment to teaching that the community pediatricians show for residents and medical students, as well as in the coordination of care and consultation provided by the Vermont Children's Hospital to rural populations both via telemedicine and in person. Located in Burlington, Vermont, the children's hospital is now part of the larger Vermont Health Network that includes regional hospitals and primary care practices throughout Vermont.

Approximately 60% of Vermonters live in rural counties, and although most children in the state live in Chittenden County (the most populous county in Vermont), children of all ages and developmental stages live throughout all of Vermont and require access to high-quality pediatric care. In addition, the catchment area for the University of Vermont Children's Hospital is wide-ranging, inclusive of much of upstate New York (sometimes a 5-hour drive to Burlington), as well as the entire state of Vermont.

As the sole training program for pediatricians in the state, the University of Vermont Children's Hospital's Pediatric Residency Program holds itself accountable to promote a sustainable workforce of pediatricians in the state. Most American Board of Pediatrics-certified pediatric subspecialists report working primarily in an urban setting (76%), with 20% practicing primarily in suburban settings and 3% practicing primarily in rural settings. Comparatively, approximately 19% of children (aged 17 years and younger) live in rural areas. Among pediatricians who completed training in 2012 through 2021, nearly 31% of subspecialists (on average) report practicing in a medically underserved area. Furthermore, on average, nearly 60% of subspecialists are practicing in the state where they completed their training.[10] Because medical residents as a whole favor postresidency career placement within the catchment of their training hospital, it is hoped that prioritizing recruitment, focused training, and retention of rural medicine providers will address health care gaps for Vermont's children.

In response to these concerns, the Vermont residency program has developed a "Rural Medicine Concentration" pathway through its 3-year categorical pediatric residency program, piloted in 2022, and designed to recruit and provide specialized training for pediatricians to serve rural and underserved populations in their future careers with a focus on retention of pediatricians in the State of Vermont. This program is advertised to prospective applicants to recruit incoming residents who are interested in caring for rural populations. The concentration allows house staff to tailor their experiences to best prepare them for a future in rural practice. The program also focuses on mentorship to provide the resident with the specialized insight and career guidance from an experienced rural physician. Exposure to rural medical practices may also promote retention of pediatricians in these areas around the state.

As part of the rural medicine concentration, residents will complete required rotations from the options as depicted in **Box 2**. They communicate with the program director in crafting their individualized education plan, and chief resident when planning schedules, to assure that requirements are met and are tailored toward effective preparation for future career aspirations.

The rural concentration is dependent on relationships with established faculty in rural practice who play a crucial role for the recruitment and retention of pediatric trainees into careers in rural regions. Mentors guide trainees in setting and reaching goals for professional growth, educational experiences, and clinical competence. Pairing residents with rural pediatricians promotes realistic discussion surrounding the benefits and challenges of rural practice. Connections made through mentorship also provide opportunities for community engagement and networking around the state and region to assist in job placement following graduate medical training. Mentors often serve as long-term supports and colleagues for early career pediatricians entering rural medicine.

At the initiation of entrance into the Rural Concentration, residents identify possible career mentors with the assistance of the rotation director and program leadership.

Box 2
University of Vermont Children's Hospital Residency Program rural concentration

PGY-1 Year

- Advocacy Rotation
  - Focus advocacy project on areas of rural well-being and health
  - Prioritize community opportunities that address needs of rural populations

PGY-2 Year

- Community Pediatrics
  - Prioritize rural rotation location (as established for Rural and Underserved Pediatrics rotation or complete nontraditional application for novel location)

PGY-3 Year

- Rural and Underserved Pediatrics
  - Select location from established clinical sites in Vermont or complete nontraditional elective application for a novel location
  - Rotations out of state include connections with practices in Montana and Arizona
- Electives (residents choose at least 2 sites for block rotations and discuss with Program Director)
  - Central Valley Physicians Hospital in Plattsburgh, New York
  - Central Vermont Medical Center in Montpelier, Vermont
  - Advanced newborn nursery
  - Neonatal delivery room selective
  - Procedure elective (nontraditional)
  - Anesthesia elective with training in the comfort zone (behavioral interventions for children undergoing painful procedures)
- Each of the regional hospital locations include clinical experience in the emergency department, newborn nursery, and primary care

Assigned faculty advisors (done by program leadership at the beginning of training) may also facilitate connections with community mentors. Residents feel empowered to directly connect with potential mentors and can seek to form relationships with the following:

- Site leaders of established Rural and Underserved Pediatrics practices
- Designated faculty at network sites in Vermont and New York
- University of Vermont Children's Hospital resident alumni practicing in rural regions
- Pediatricians identified by residents based on individual goals and experiences (such as from current/prior/future community, medical school, preresidency employment, and so forth)

At the completion of the Rural Health Concentration upon graduation from the residency program, each resident produces one "deliverable" to be reviewed with the rotation director. Listed below are some possible options for rural health deliverables, but other projects are considered with approval by the rotation director:

- Longitudinal advocacy project with rural basis
- Quality improvement project focused on rural health or communities
- Reflective assessment and review of health and associated resources in a specific rural community in Vermont
- Educational presentation on rural health topic at Professor Rounds and/or for students or community practice groups

In association with the Rural Concentration, but open to all residents in the University of Vermont Children's Hospital program, focused didactics within the resident teaching schedule with a 3-year rolling curriculum with 3 cycles include the following:

1. Injury prevention: Traumatic brain injury prevention, water safety, car seat safety, childproofing
2. Special populations: Amish health and culture, Abenaki and Wabanaki culture, migrant farmworker health, children with medical complexity
3. Rural health considerations: Wilderness medicine, agricultural health, addiction medicine

To date, the rural concentration program has successfully placed one pediatric resident into practice in rural Vermont in the fall of 2023, with a second expected to graduate in 2025.

In terms of data over the last 15 years, the UVMCH program has produced 100 pediatricians. Of those, 44% pursued primary care after their training (12% of those choosing primary care entering practice as hospitalists without additional fellowship training), and 56% pursued fellowship (**Fig. 3**).

Of the 44 residents that chose primary care, 22 (50%) chose to practice in a rural setting as their first job after residency, with 17% of them providing rural hospitalist care. Of those residents who pursued fellowship after graduation, 5 residents entered subspecialty care in a rural setting.

Although the UVMCH immediate community in Burlington, Vermont is not considered rural, the authors are delighted that 12 graduates who went on to fellowship over the past 15 years are now members of the faculty. The authors have trained and retained 16 residents into primary care pediatrics in Vermont, 12 of those being placed in rural settings. More impressively, 100% of the total number of residents choosing to practice rural pediatrics are either in that same first job or in a different practice that is still in a rural setting.

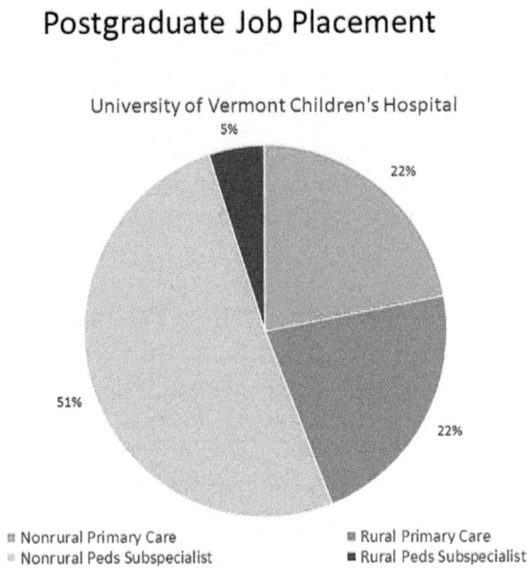

Fig. 3. University of Vermont Children's Hospital pediatric residency program postgraduate job placement.

Children's Hospital at Dartmouth–Hitchcock

The pediatric residency program at Dartmouth–Hitchcock/Mary Hitchcock Memorial Hospital was accredited in 1955 and remains the only pediatric training program in New Hampshire. Graduates of the program practice as primary care providers throughout northern New England, and there is a strong history of graduates entering pediatric subspecialty training.

The pediatric training program's primary location is at the Children's Hospital at Dartmouth–Hitchcock (CHaD) in Lebanon, New Hampshire and is affiliated with The Geisel School of Medicine at Dartmouth College. In addition to the Pediatric Residency Program, a Neonatal–Perinatal Fellowship program was established in 1992, and since then, has produced neonatologists practicing in New Hampshire and northern New England as well as across the country. Dartmouth–Hitchcock Medical Center is an academic medical center located in a rural setting, and as a result, all aspects of clinical training occurs in a rural setting, with the town of Lebanon, New Hampshire having a population of approximately 14,000, with close to 20,000 residents in the region.

In contrast to Maine and Vermont's population, approximately 70% of New Hampshire's population is located in the 3 southernmost counties of the state, with 30% of the population living in the remaining rural counties (which account for approximately two-thirds of the total area of the state). As a result, most pediatric patients and families travel up to 2 hours from across New Hampshire and Vermont to receive their care.

There is not a formal rural training track or rotation at CHaD; however, all pediatric residents complete rotations in Community Pediatrics and Advocacy, run by the Boyle Community Pediatrics Program. Established in 1997 by a concerned parent and her child's doctor, the program was initially focused on the care of both chronically ill children and their families. The driver for developing the program was the recognition that even seriously ill children often have only brief stays in the hospital and that most of the care happens at home and within the community. Because these children came and went so quickly, many pediatric residents had limited understanding of the emotional, financial, and social difficulties families with chronically ill children face. In addition, residents were not aware of what resources the community had to help families in need. The goal of this program was to train medical students and residents to practice family-centered care and look beyond the disease they were treating, resulting in healthier patients and less-stressed families. The program was named for pediatrician William Boyle, who for 35 years has been a leader in both medical education at Dartmouth and compassionate care for children and families.

First-year residents participate in a longitudinal community pediatrics rotation, which exposes them to the resources and services used by patients in both New Hampshire and Vermont, and senior residents rotate in 3-week blocks in both their second and third year of training. In the block rotations, senior residents are embedded in a rural pediatric practice (currently all participating practices are run by graduates of the pediatric residency program at CHaD). In addition to block rotations, several of the community pediatric practices host a resident longitudinally as part of their continuity clinic during all 3 years of training. In addition to the clinical experiences in the Community Pediatrics rotations, the advocacy curriculum is also embedded in the rotation to further highlight the critical role of advocacy in the rural population. The community pediatrics rotations and advocacy education are embedded in the comprehensive ambulatory pediatric curriculum, as depicted in **Box 3**.

In addition to the rural clinical experiences during the Community Pediatrics and Advocacy rotations, the inpatient experiences at a rural academic medical center have unique components that enhance resident education. As mentioned previously, most patients treated at CHaD live in a rural setting, and residents are exposed to the resource needs for rural families that are different from those in urban settings (ie, ability to travel distances for medical care, whether acute or in follow-up) and have early exposure to medical transport needs and decision making done by attendings. Many patients may present to critical access hospitals, and the pediatric hospitalists, PICU and NICU attendings all provide support to providers caring for children while transport is en route. In addition, there is a robust neonatal telehealth system that residents are able to participate in with NICU attendings in the support of referring providers in neonatal resuscitation and stabilization. Residents also develop a strong level of autonomy during their training, with excellent opportunities for procedural experience and leadership in clinical decision making and code events that might be less common in a residency program with a large number of fellowship programs.

In a small rural pediatric training program, residents work directly with pediatric subspecialist attendings clinically and on scholarly activity, and this close mentorship results in residents applying to pediatric subspecialty fellowship programs annually. Since 2008, 105 residents have graduated from the pediatric residency program, with 48% entering general pediatric practice (outpatient or pediatric hospitalist without fellowship training), and 52% completed pediatric subspecialty fellowship training (**Fig. 4**). Of the residents entering practice directly from residency, 33% practice in a rural setting and 66% practice in a suburban or urban setting. For the residents completing subspecialty fellowship, 20% practice in their subspecialty in a rural setting, including residents who have chosen to return to the authors' institution to practice postfellowship training. In addition, the trend over the last 15 years has been an increase per year of the number of residents entering pediatric subspecialty fellowship after completing residency, which is interesting in an era when there is an overall decrease in the number of pediatric residents applying for subspecialty

Box 3
Children's Hospital at Dartmouth–Hitchcock Residency Program comprehensive ambulatory pediatric curriculum

PGY-1 Year

- Continuity Clinics—completed in half-day sessions in "Y week" rotations
  - One resident per year completes their continuity clinic experience at a rural pediatrics practice
- Acute Care Pediatrics—completed in half-day sessions in "Y week" rotations
- Community Pediatrics and Advocacy Rotation—longitudinal experience in one half-day session during each "Y week" rotation
  - Site visits to community services for patients
  - Experiences in rural pediatric practices
  - Focused introduction and education on advocacy

PGY-2 Year

- Continuity Clinics—completed in half-day sessions in "Y week" rotations
  - One resident per year completes their continuity clinic experience at a rural pediatrics practice
- Acute Care Pediatrics—completed in half-day sessions in "Y week" rotations
- Community Pediatrics and Advocacy Rotation
  - Completed in a rural community pediatrics practice during a 3-week rotation
  - Advocacy project design exercise
  - Educational presentation to clinical site

PGY-3 Year

- Continuity Clinics—completed in half-day sessions in "Y week" rotations
  - One resident per year completes their continuity clinic experience at a rural pediatrics practice
- Acute Care Pediatrics—completed in half-day sessions in "Y week" rotations
- Community Pediatrics and Advocacy Rotation
  - Individualized experience per resident during a 3-week rotation
    - Rural community pediatrics practice experience
    - Rural community hospitalist experience
    - Advocacy rotation focused on an advocacy project

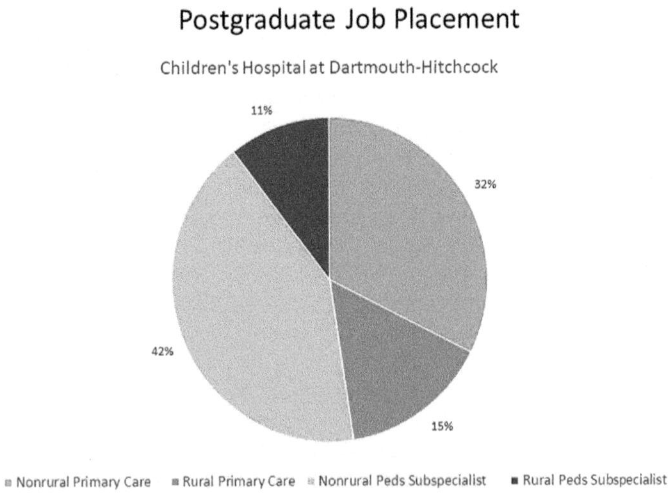

Fig. 4. CHaD pediatric residency program postgraduate job placement.

fellowship training. Although this may be multifactorial, a contributing factor could be that in a small rural training program, the opportunities for procedures, leadership, and graduated autonomy in clinical decision making and close mentorship from subspecialty faculty are driving forces for residents to choose fellowship training.

DISCUSSION

The authors' experience with 3 small pediatric residency programs in Northern New England without formal rural tracks demonstrates that exposure to rural medicine during residency training leads to a greater number of learners pursing postgraduate practice in rural pediatric medicine. Graduate data comparing primary care versus pediatric subspecialty training as well as rural versus suburban or urban practice settings are consistent and similar across the authors' training programs. This highlights that training programs that naturally include greater exposure to rural medicine during training leads to more residents choosing careers in rural medicine.

As noted in the introduction as well as by each of the author's programs, the pediatric subspecialty workforce is shrinking, and it is important for all training programs to produce graduates interested in pursuing subspecialty fellowships as well as primary care. Residents training in all 3 of the authors' programs have a greater degree of autonomy in caring for patients than often experienced in larger pediatric residency training programs that also have pediatric fellowship trainees. This autonomy and direct contact with subspecialty leadership results in approximately half of the residents in all 3 of the authors' programs to pursue fellowship training.

In addition to rural medicine opportunities, the authors' programs all include a strong education in advocacy, crucial to the role of a pediatrician practicing in any setting and especially to those practicing in a rural setting. In addition to the advocacy curricula in each of the authors' programs, in 2018 the 3 programs joined together to create the Northern New England Advocacy Collaborative (NNEAC) with the goals of providing education, providing collaboration, and building relationships across the training programs and state AAP chapters. A key component to NNEAC is the focus on the needs of patients in rural settings, as well as education of the trainees on the importance of providing advocacy on behalf of their rural patients and families.

SUMMARY

Training pediatricians to successfully practice in a rural setting is crucial, and the embedded exposure to rural medicine in residency training programs is one model resulting in both primary care and pediatric subspecialists choosing to practice in a rural setting. The opportunities for autonomy, procedural training, and advocacy training help to prepare future rural pediatricians for practice.

DISCLOSURE

The authors have nothing to disclose.

REFERENCES

1. Attracting the next generation of physicians to rural medicine. AAMC News. Available at: https://www.aamc.org/news/attracting-next-generation-physicians-rural-medicine. [Accessed 16 February 2024].
2. Skinner L, Staiger DO, Auerbach DI, et al. Implications of an Aging Rural Physician Workforce. N Engl J Med 2019;381(4):299–301.

3. Shipman SA, Wendling A, Jones KC, et al. The Decline In Rural Medical Students: A Growing Gap In Geographic Diversity Threatens The Rural Physician Workforce. Health Aff (Millwood) 2019;38(12):2011–8.
4. Lavergne MR, Goldsmith LJ, Grudniewicz A, et al. Practice patterns among early-career primary care (ECPC) physicians and workforce planning implications: protocol for a mixed methods study. BMJ Open 2019;9(9):e030477.
5. Russell DJ, Wilkinson E, Petterson S, et al. Family Medicine Residencies: How Rural Training Exposure in GME Is Associated With Subsequent Rural Practice. J Grad Med Educ 2022;14(4):441–50.
6. Elma A, Nasser M, Yang L, et al. Medical education interventions influencing physician distribution into underserved communities: a scoping review. Hum Resour Health 2022;20(1):31.
7. Coe CL, Baker HM, Byerley JS, et al. Fully Integrated Readiness for Service Training (FIRST): An Accelerated Medical Training Program for Rural and Underserved North Carolina. Acad Med 2021;96(10):1436–40.
8. Longenecker RL, Andrilla CHA, Jopson AD, et al. Pipelines to Pathways: Medical School Commitment to Producing a Rural Workforce. J Rural Health 2021;37(4):723–33.
9. Enhancing pediatric workforce diversity and providing culturally effective pediatric care: implications for practice, education, and policy making. Pediatrics 2013;132(4):e1105–16.
10. National Academies of Sciences E, Medicine, Division of B. The future pediatric subspecialty physician workforce: meeting the needs of infants, children, and adolescents. National Academies Press (US) Copyright 2023 by the National Academy of Sciences. All rights reserved.; 2023.